W0116037

Pharmacovigilance in the European Union

Michael Kaeding · Julia Schmälter
Christoph Klika

Pharmacovigilance in the European Union

Practical Implementation across Member States

OPEN

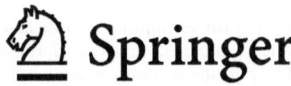

Prof. Dr. Michael Kaeding
Julia Schmälter
Christoph Klika

Universität Duisburg-Essen
Duisburg, Deutschland

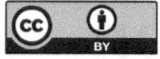

ISBN 978-3-658-17275-6   ISBN 978-3-658-17276-3   (eBook)
DOI 10.1007/978-3-658-17276-3

Library of Congress Control Number: 2017932440

Lektorat: Jan Treibel

Printed on acid-free paper

This Springer imprint is published by Springer Nature
The registered company is Springer Fachmedien Wiesbaden GmbH
The registered company address is: Abraham-Lincoln-Str. 46, 65189 Wiesbaden, Germany

Contents

Abbreviations

ÄAAS	Ärzteausschuss Arzneimittelsicherheit (Germany)
ADR	Adverse Drug Reaction
AFSSAPS	Agence Française de Sécurité Sanitaire des Produits de Santé (France)
AGRIFISH	Agriculture and Fisheries (Council))
AkdÄ	Arzneimittelkommission der Deutschen Ärzteschaft (Germany)
AMK	Arzneimittelkommission der Deutschen Apotheker (Germany)
ANSM	Agence Nationale de Securité du Medicament et des Produits de Santé (France)
BfArM	Bundesinstitut für Arzneimittel und Medizinprodukte (Germany)
CHMP	Committee for Medicinal Products for Human Use
CMPh	Co-ordination Group for Mutual Recognition and Decentralised procedures – Human
CRPV	Centre Régionaux de Pharmacovigilance (France)
DG	Directorate General (European Commission)
EBGM	Empirical Bayes Geometric Mean (Method)
EMA	European Medicines Agency
ENVI	Environment, Public Health and Food Safety (European Parliament)
EP	European Parliament
EPSCO	Employment, Social Policy, Health and Consumer Affairs (Council)
EU	European Union
FPD	French Pharmacovigilance Database
Fimea	Lääkealan Turvallisuus- Ja Kehittämiskeskus (Finland)
GDP	Good Distribution Practice
GIS	Główny Inspektorat Sanitarny (Poland)
GMP	Good Manufacturing Practice
GROWTH	Directorate General Internal Market, Industry, Entrepreneurship and SMEs (European Commission)
GVP	Good Pharmacovigilance Practice

HCP	Healthcare Professional
ICSR	Individual Case Safety Report
IMCO	Internal market and Consumer Protection (European Parlaiment)
INFARMED	Autoridade Nacional do Medicamento e Produtos de Saúde (Portugal)
IT	Information Technology
ITRE	Industry, research and Energy (European Parliament)
MAH	Marketing Authorisation Holder
MDSO	Medical Device Safety Officer
MHRA	Medicines and Healthcare Products Regulatory Agency (United Kingdom)
MSO	Medical Safety Officer
NCA	National Competent Authority
NHS	National Health Service (United Kingdom)
NIM	National Implementing Measure
PASS	Post-Authorisation Safety Study
PEI	Paul-Ehrlich-Institut (Germany)
PHAGRO	Bundesverband des Pharmazeutischen Großhandels (Germany)
PRAC	Pharmacovigilance Risk Assessment Committee
SANTE	Directorate General Health and Food Safety (European Commission)
SCOPE	Strengthening Collaboration for Operating Pharmacovigilance in Europe
THL	Terveyden-Ja Hyvinvoinnin Laitos (National Institute for Health and Welfare, Finland)
URF	Unidade Regional de Farmacovigiláncia (Portugal)
URPL	Urząd Rejestracji Produktów Leczniczych, Wyrobów Medycznych i Produktów Biobójczych (Poland)
WHO	World Health Organisation
WIS	Wojewodzki Inspektorat Sanitarny (Poland)
YCC	Yellow Card Centre (United Kingdom)

List of Tables, Figures and Boxes

Preface

This implementation assessment, "Pharmacovigilance in the EU: Practical Implementation across Member States" is the result of intensive teamwork. The assessment was commissioned by AbbVie, directed by Dr Michael Kaeding and managed by Julia Schmälter. In addition, the group of collaborators included Christoph Klika, Roxana Dürsch, Annika Körner, Stella Malliara and Charline Ulrich.

"Pharmacovigilance in the EU: Practical Implementation across Member States" comes at a time when Europe faces rising populism and Euroscepticism, and a time when Europe needs to find effective responses to pressing European and global issues – in short, to develop a new narrative. Europe has to deliver by reaching out to its Member States and must prove more than ever its added value. Non-compliance with EU rules implies legal uncertainty and hampers the European regulatory framework in which citizens live and businesses operate. In addition, non-compliance frustrates further European integration, including the free movement of people, goods, services and capital, and potentially jeopardizes market competitiveness, social standards, national growth and employment performance across Europe.

Our implementation assessment studies the practical implementation of pharmacovigilance across Europe. European pharmacovigilance has been geared towards the detection of adverse reactions to medicinal products to ensure public health through product safety and to provide medicinal products with a high level of efficacy.

The research for this assessment would have been impossible without fruitful discussions and collaborations with colleagues and implementation scholars during the 10 months of investigation. Some of our thoughts that eventually turned into chapters were presented at conferences: the IRUN compliance workshop, "Non-compliance with EU Regulatory Norms, Rules and Values" at the University of Duisburg-Essen, the ECSA-C 11th Biennial Conference in Halifax, the ECPR Pan-European Conference on the European Union in Trento, the ECPR General Conference at the Charles University of Prague, and the GAfPA Patient Advocacy and Safety Conference in Brussels.

Furthermore, this assessment would have been impossible without the support of our interview partners. Many thanks to all those we met in Berlin, Bonn, Brussels, Helsinki, Lisbon, London, Liverpool, Paris, Reims and Warsaw, who contributed by kindly agreeing to give up their valuable time to participate in in-depth interviews conducted by the Duisburg-Essen pharmacovigilance research team. Moreover, the team is grateful to Monika Bähtz and Peter Staniczek for their administrative support and to Elizabeth Meyer zu Heringdorf for her linguistic expertise.

Finally, the views expressed in this implementation assessment are those of its authors, and these views neither reflect those of their institution of employment nor its staff. The authors are solely responsible for any mistakes or inaccuracies.

Dr Michael Kaeding, Julia Schmälter and Christoph Klika
Brussels and Duisburg, December 2016

Introduction

1.1   Background and Terms of Reference

Healthcare is a major component of the contemporary welfare state, and thus ensuring public health through product safety is a substantive public concern.

It is universally accepted that all medicines might produce adverse drug reactions (ADRs) during the course of their normal therapeutic use (Belton and the European Pharmacovigilance Research Group 1997). In order to ensure post-marketing authorisation safety, all suspected ADRs must be reported in an accurate and timely manner.

Due to the use of living cells, biological medicinal products (so-called biologicals) pose a specific challenge for pharmacovigilance and the accurate reporting of ADRs for mainly four reasons: restrictions in clinical trials, sensitivity to changes in the manufacturing process, reporting of batch numbers and the establishment of valid causality assessments.

For these reasons, the timely and accurate reporting of ADRs is particularly important when it comes to the use of biological products. In order to ensure the correct and timely attribution of adverse events to the correct biological product and batch, the availability of information such as the international non-proprietary name, the brand name, the company's name and the batch number are extremely important.

The former European Union (EU) pharmaceuticals legislation (Directive 2001/83/EC) underwent an extensive reform process since 2006, which resulted in a new Directive (2010/84/EU) and Regulation (No 1235/2010) in 2010, bringing about significant changes to pharmacovigilance in general and ADR reporting in particular.

The new legislation, in force since July 2012, strengthens the monitoring of medicinal products in general and biologicals in particular to ensure public health through product safety. The new legislation is geared towards the detection of adverse reactions to medicinal products that have been authorised for marketing, and it consists of activities and methods for detecting, assessing, informing on and preventing ADRs.

In August 2016 the European Commission (Commission) published its assessment of the new EU pharmacovigilance legislation. The assessment consists of two documents, namely the Commission Report titled "Pharmacovigilance-related Activities of Member States and the EMA Concerning Medical Products for Human Use (2012-2014)" and the related Commission staff working document. The first document, an eight-page report, mainly explains the role of the relevant actors involved (Member States, EMA and the Commission) and the main activities related to pharmacovigilance. Further, the report provides statistics on the numbers of pharmacovigilance-related reports and activities between 2012 and 2014 (such as ADR reports), showing that the situation in Europe has been steadily improving since the adoption of the new pharmacovigilance legislation. The Commission staff working document is more elaborate (54 pages) and includes additional information on activities related to ADR reporting, such as improvements in strengthening patient involvement or awareness-raising campaigns (European Commission 2016, 10-12).

Both Commission documents, however, only scratch the surface and do not go into further detail about the overall day-to-day functioning of the pharmacovigilance systems in single Member States, the remaining challenges, or factors that might impede or incentivise ADR reporting. Most important, they lack country-specific and detailed information about the ADR reporting of biologicals.

This also holds for the work conducted by the three-year Joint Action, called the "Strengthening Collaboration for Operating Pharmacovigilance in Europe" (SCOPE, 2013-2016). Funded by the Consumers, Health and Food Executive Agency,[1] this collaborative joint action was created to support effective implementation of the pharmacovigilance reform. SCOPE aims at delivering practical tools to and guidance for nation regulatory authorities to ensure the consistent development of pharmacovigilance systems across Europe, including training in key aspects of pharmacovigilance and tools and templates that aim to support best practices across Europe. SCOPE was divided into eight separate work packages, one of which focused on improvements in ADR reporting.

Overall, SCOPE offers a useful source of information for horizontal aspects of national pharmacovigilance systems in Europe. It provides a fuller general understanding of, and develops best practices in, reporting mechanisms for ADRs.

However, SCOPE pays little attention to biologicals. Moreover, its survey data does not allow tracing back country-specific information. Therefore, SCOPE does

---

1   Executive agencies in the EU are created by the Commission to support the implementation of specific programmes, inter alia, in the area of public health.

not contribute to a Member State-specific understanding of reporting mechanisms for ADRs regarding biologicals.

In summary, our study focuses on the ADR reporting of biologicals and on specific EU Member States representing various types of healthcare systems across Europe. Assessing the timely transposition and accurate implementation of the European pharmacovigilance framework as described in Directive 2010/84/EU, this report aims at identifying major drivers impeding and incentivising appropriate ADR reporting in Europe. Our assessment offers a rich and detailed account of ADR reporting systems across individual Member States, identifying perceived challenges and best practices in order to formulate recommendations on the necessary conditions for robust and effective systems ensuring accurate identification and rapid traceability of biological medicines.

1.2 Methodology: Selection of Countries

Assessing medical services has become a political issue throughout the industrialised world. The utilisation of health services is influenced by the activities of physicians, hospitals, professional associations, interest groups, legislative chambers and administrators. Furthermore, it is influenced by the competition of rival ideologies. Thus, systems can be centralised or decentralised, or possibly fragmented in a recentralised state.

Therefore, our research strategy for the EU pharmacovigilance implementation project goes beyond single-country studies. Its geographic scope covers six areas, distinguishing between ideal systems – namely, state healthcare systems and societal healthcare systems (as well as various permutations of mixed systems thereof):

- United Kingdom (ideal-type state healthcare system)
- Finland (state-based mixed type)
- Poland (state-based mixed type)
- France (state-based mixed type)
- Portugal (societal-based mixed type)
- Germany (societal-based mixed type)

Essentially, there are three responsibilities in healthcare: first, the financing of health services through taxation, social insurance contributions or private means; second, the provision of healthcare which can be carried out in state-run facilities by state-based actors, in societal-based facilities, or in private for-profit facilities by private actors; and third, the regulation by these actors of the various aspects of financing and provision (Moran 1999; Burau and Blank 2004). Taken together, the financing, service provision and regulation of healthcare are three key dimensions along which different groups of actors may take on numerous roles and exhibit varying levels of engagement. However, in "real" medical care systems, the "state", "societal" and "private" elements tend to coexist alongside each other in all three dimensions. Therefore, when analysing changes over time, the mix within categories is taken into consideration.

Based on uniform features across all dimensions of healthcare, we identified three instances of ideal types. These types comprise state healthcare systems, in which financing, service provision and regulation are carried out by state actors and institutions; societal healthcare systems, in which societal actors take on the responsibility of healthcare financing, provision and regulation; and finally private healthcare systems, in which all three dimensions fall under the auspices of market actors.

In total, six empirical cases illustrate different arrangements for governing the medical care sector and their associated political problems. The United Kingdom, Finland, Poland, France, Portugal and Germany have different public traditions concerning the ratio of individual versus collective responsibility for social welfare in general and medical care in particular.

Given their respective histories and patterns of development, Finland and the United Kingdom have well-developed prototypes of organisational and political arrangements. The United Kingdom is highly centralised and its National Health Service (NHS) is directly financed by the central government out of general tax revenues. Significant changes have taken place intra-dimensionally such that there has been an internal shift of levels. The introduction of an internal market in the United Kingdom has not led to a replacement of the state as the main regulator; however, the United Kingdom has created some space for self-regulation through NHS trusts. Finland, although a unitary state, has granted important financial and organisational roles to local authorities, and it has decentralised many health-related functions to regional levels.

Germany can be characterised by predominantly social-insurance-based regulation and financing combined with a high and increasing share of private healthcare provision. In addition, the current growth of state intervention in Germany even enlarges the distance to the societal-based ideal type.

Poland is exemplary for Central and Eastern Europe which has changed from socialist healthcare systems to social health insurance systems (Dubois and McKee 2004) and is currently characterised by comparatively weak social insurance systems actors and a high proportion of healthcare being provided in public hospitals.

Despite the low level of tax funding, Poland can still be classified as the state-based mixed type, and only a strengthening of corporate social insurance actors would lead to a real system change.

Southern European countries changed from a social insurance type to a national-health-service type in the late 1970s and early 1980s (Guillén and Matsaganis 2000). In contrast to France, however, Portugal maintained elements of the former social health insurance scheme and is characterised by weak public authorities (Cabiedes and Guillén 2001).[2] Despite the weakness of state authorities, the changes of the 1970s and 1980s seem to represent a system shift from a societal-based mixed type towards a state-based mixed type (Wendt et al. 2009).

1.3   Methodology: Research Strategy

The primary assessment program involves a range of research methodologies that are both quantitative and qualitative. Based on a mainly threefold methodological approach, including qualitative, quantitative and benchmarking methods, the findings and recommendations have emerged from a most appropriate, sequential desk and field research process, benchmarking, and interviews across the six selected Member States, national (hospital) pharmacist associations, national regulatory agencies, and those administering systems for post-marketing safety surveillance of biologicals, including spontaneous reporting systems and external stakeholders.

The research strategy for the EU pharmacovigilance implementation project comprises five key stages, as outlined below and detailed in the following paragraphs:

- Desk-based analysis
- Document research
- Key informant interviews
- In-depth field research
- Benchmarking

Desk-based analysis. There is a vast literature on pharmacovigilance dealing with incentives of healthcare professionals to report ADRs. This literature was crucial for developing analytical categories for both desk-based and field-based research. However, given that this literature is part of the health sciences, it is concerned

---

2   Spain, in contrast, has experienced reforms of the medical care sector which means that it no longer has a societal-type system.

primarily with individual factors of ADR reporting, and it necessarily neglects political implications at the systems level. Furthermore, research designs are mostly based on surveys conducted in single case studies, and thus deal with countries in isolation. Extending on this literature, the six empirical case studies, based on varying organisational and political arrangements, allow for a better contextualisation of ADR reporting.

A comparative case study, with cases selected on an ideal-type health system, provides for added benefit to the existing literature.

Document research. Assessing the transposition of the European pharmacovigilance framework involved conducting a documentation review. This first phase helped collect useful information on the timely and correct transposition, management and governance of compliance with Directive 2010/84/EU across all EU-28 Member States. Information on the EU pharmacovigilance Directive was taken from the official legal database of the EU, which covers all Member State legislation and provides publication references regarding Member States' national provisions to enact EU legislation. Because Member States often transpose EU legislation by using more than one national transposing instrument, we recorded all transposing instruments that were indicated to the Commission until March 2016. Because the recorded measures do not indicate whether the national implementation process is complete, a second step was put in place.

Key informant interviews. It is essential that practitioners, industry and regulators participate in the reporting of suspected ADRs in order to ensure accurate traceability back to the manufacturer. Consequently, formal schemes were established in every country to enable healthcare professionals and the public to report ADRs.

This step involved a series of in-depth interviews which were carried out, either face-to-face or by telephone, with different stakeholder groups to map the national pharmacovigilance systems. We developed a list of potential interview partners who would be relevant for the study, and from this list of stakeholders, we conducted 33 key informant interviews with executives, healthcare professionals, the industry and patient organisations between April and September 2016.

On the basis of these interviews, the country chapters mapping the respective national pharmacovigilance systems were finalised and a first set of perceived best practices and challenges was drafted.

In-depth field research. The third step in assessing the European pharmacovigilance framework as described in Directive 2010/84/EU involved in-depth study and visits to the six selected countries. This step also helped us compare the different national systems and develop recommendations.

Simultaneously, monitoring data provided in documents, websites and reports reflecting the current state of play of academic literature was performed. This has included collecting details on the number and features of adverse drug reporting, incurred by the following studies:

- Andrews, E., Moore, N. (eds) (2014). *Mann's Pharmacovigilance*. Wiley-Blackwell Oxford.
- Drozd et al. (2014). *Biosimilar Drugs – Automatic Substitution Regulations Review. Polish ISPOR Chapter's Therapeutic Programmes and Pharmaceutical Care (TPPC) Task Force Report.* Journal of Health Policy 1: 52-57.
- European Commission (2016). *Pharmacovigilance Related Activities of Member States and the European Medicines Agency Concerning Medicinal Products for Human Use (2012-2014)*, COM(2016) 498 final, Brussels, 08.08.2016.
- SCOPE (2016). *Work Package 4 – ADR Collection.*
- Vermeer et al. (2015). *Traceability of Biologicals: Present Challenges in Pharmacovigilance.* Expert Opinion on Drug Safety 14 (1).

Benchmarking. Benchmarking analysis included a comparative assessment of cases highlighting perceived best practices versus perceived challenges in developing national systems, allowing for the identification of biologicals by brand name and batch number.

By utilising these comparative materials, we were able to see the relative strengths as well as the chronic problems of the EU pharmacovigilance system. Drawing on desk- and field-based research, these findings complement and add significantly to primarily theoretical discussions about the system (see Borg et al. 2015; Calvo and Zuñiga 2014). The research distinguishes the malleable from the inevitable in health-related decision-making across Europe and thereby suggests the constrained nature of policy options in Western democratic societies.

1.4   Summary of Evidence

This study presents our findings and conclusions that were formed by assessing all of the elements in the cumulative process described here. Additional interviews were conducted to validate the emerging conclusions that we reached from the benchmarking analysis and field and desk research. We weighed all evidence equally, except when the evidence was clearly unrepresentative or not credible. In cases where we do not provide specific evidence to support a finding or conclusion, it is because we have combined the evidence to present a summary conclusion. The recommendations are based on our own analysis.

1.5   Implementation Assessment Structure

The main purpose of this EU pharmacovigilance implementation study is to present the findings of the comparative assessment of six national ADR reporting systems for biologicals and to outline recommendations for future action. After having put the implementation assessment into context and taking into account the complexity of the study through a threefold methodological approach, we determined six important goals, corresponding to the following structure of the manuscript:

- Chapter 2: Pharmacovigilance. This chapter outlines the fundamentals of pharmacovigilance with a particular emphasis on the role of healthcare professionals when it comes to ADR reporting. The chapter also explains why pharmacovigilance is specifically important regarding biologicals.
- Chapter 3: The EU Pharmacovigilance System. This chapter outlines the main objectives of pharmaceutical regulation in the EU, tracing the developments in terms of pharmacovigilance. It identifies the complex network of EU actors and presents the key features of the current EU pharmacovigilance system. In addition, this chapter also presents in detail the reform of Directive 2010/84/EU and how it aims to facilitate ADR reporting in general and biologicals in particular.
- Chapter 4: Timely and Correct Transposition of Pharmacovigilance across Member States. This chapter offers a first assessment of the timeliness of national transposition processes for all EU Member States and shows that many countries have a serious transposition problem in their national pharmacovigilance systems. Unfortunately, it appears that the EU transposition deficit is more than just a statistical illusion. Almost 85 percent of the national transposition instruments are not transposed on time, and in fact are delayed up to more than two years.

Cross-country variance is significant, and the difference between the laggards (Denmark and Slovenia) and the champions (Cyprus, Romania, Sweden, Estonia, the United Kingdom and Ireland) is remarkable.

- Chapter 5: <u>Practical Implementation of Pharmacovigilance in Six Member States</u>. The aim of this chapter is threefold. First, it offers in-depth explanations of the ADR reporting systems, and describes relevant tasks and actors involved in the United Kingdom, Finland, France, Poland, Portugal and Germany. Second, it presents remaining challenges and best practices for each case as perceived by the interview partners. Third, it provides first recommendations on how to improve the existing systems in order to improve ADR reporting and help ensure public health.
- Chapter 6: <u>Challenges and Best Practices in Perspective</u>. This chapter offers an analysis of the findings presented in Chapter 5. Here, the six different ADR reporting systems are directly compared and the remaining challenges and best practices put into perspective.
- Chapter 7: <u>Conclusions and Recommendations</u>. This chapter summarises the main findings that have emerged from the EU pharmacovigilance implementation assessment. On the basis of the results, the chapter outlines specific recommendations in relation to the provisions of Article 2 of Directive 2010/84/EU. Drawing on these specific recommendations, the chapter puts forward general recommendations in the context of national healthcare systems, suggesting the constrained nature of policy options in Western democratic societies. This policy context is crucial for understanding questions about pharmacovigilance and its challenges for practical implementation across Member States.

References

Andrews, E., Moore, N. (2014). *Mann's Pharmacovigilance*. Wiley-Blackwell, Oxford.

Belton, K. J. and the European Pharmacovigilance Group (1997). *Attitude Survey of Adverse Drug-Reaction Reporting by Health Care Professionals across the European Union*. European Journal of Pharmacology 52: 423-427.

Borg, J. J., Tanti, A., Kouvelas, D., Lungu, C., Prozynski, M., Serracino-Inglott, A., Aislaitner, G. (2015). *European Union Pharmacovigilance Capabilities: Potential for the New Legislation*. Therapeutic Advances in Drug Safety 6 (4): 120-140.

Burau, V., Blank, R. H. (2006). *Comparing Health Policy: An Assessment of Typologies of Health Systems*. Journal of Comparative Policy Analysis 8 (1): 63–76.

Cabiedes, L., Guillén, A. (2001). *Adopting and Adapting Managed Competition: Health Care Reform in Southern Europe*. Social Science and Medicine 52: 1205-1217.

Calvo, B., Zuñiga, L. (2014). *EU's New Pharmacovigilance Legislation: Considerations for Biosimilars*. Drug Safety 37: 9-18.

Drozd, M., Szkultecka-Dębek, M., Baran-Lewandowska, I. (2014). *Biosimilar Drugs – Automatic Substitution Regulations Review. Polish ISPOR Chapter's Therapeutic Programmes and Pharmaceutical Care (TPPC) Task Force Report*. Journal of Health Policy 1: 52-57.

Dubois, C.-A., McKee, M. (2004). Health and Health Care in the Candidate Countries of the European Union: Common Challenges, Different Circumstances, Diverse Policies. McKee, M., MacLehose, L., Nolte, E. (eds) (2004). *Health Policy and European Union Enlargement*. Maidenhead: Open University Press: 43-63.

European Commission (2016). *Pharmacovigilance Related Activities of Member States and the European Medicines Agency Concerning Medicinal Products for Human Use (2012-2014)*, COM(2016) 498 final, Brussels, 08.08.2016.

Guillén, A. M., Matsaganis, M. (2000). *Testing the 'Social Dumping' Hypothesis in Southern Europe: Welfare Policies in Greece and Spain During the Last 20 Years*. Journal of European Social Policy 10 (2): 120-145.

Moran, M. (1999) Governing the Health Care State: A Comparative Study of the United Kingdom, the United States and Germany. Manchester: Manchester University Press.

SCOPE (2016). *Work Package 4 – ADR Collection*.

Vermeer, N. S., Spierings, I., Mantel-Teeuwisse, A. K., Straus, S. M. J. M., Giezen, T. J., Leufkens, H. G. M., Egberts, T. C. G., De Bruin, M. L. (2015). *Traceability of Biologicals: Present Challenges in Pharmacovigilance*. Expert Opinion on Drug Safety, 14 (1).

Wendt, C., Frisina, L., Rothgang, H. (2009). *Healthcare System Types: A Conceptual Framework for Comparison*. Social Policy and Administration 43 (1): 70-90.

Pharmacovigilance 2

In this chapter, the fundamentals of pharmacovigilance are outlined with a particular emphasis on the role of healthcare professionals in reporting adverse drug reactions (ADRs). It also explains why pharmacovigilance is specifically important regarding biological medicinal products (biologicals).

2.1 Fundamentals of Pharmacovigilance

Before medicinal products are marketed, they undergo extensive risk assessment, including clinical trials. After marketing authorisation, drugs are prescribed to larger populations in medical environments that are less controlled than clinical trials. Hence, medicines might produce ADRs during normal therapeutic use, despite risk assessment during marketing authorisation (Belton and the European Pharmacovigilance Research Group 1997).

It is estimated that ADRs account for five percent of all hospital admissions and cause around 200,000 deaths per year in the European Union (EU) (European Commission 2008). Based on the estimation by the European Commission (Commission), the total cost of ADRs amounts to roughly €80 billion.

Hence, product safety is a substantive public concern and essential for public health. Patients might be harmed not only by a drug itself, but also due to the combined interaction of more than one prescribed drug. In order to prevent harm, the surveillance of medicinal products is vital and pharmacovigilance has become an important aspect of public health legislation (Johnson and Hutchinson 2015).

The World Health Organisation (WHO) defines pharmacovigilance as "the science and activities relating to the detection, assessment, understanding and prevention of adverse effects or any other medicine-related problem" (WHO 2004).

Pharmacovigilance pursues the following four general objectives (WHO 2004):

- "To improve patient care and safety in relation to the use of medicines, and all medical and paramedical interventions;
- to improve public health and safety in relation to the use of medicines;
- to contribute to the assessment of benefit, harm, effectiveness and risk of medicines, encouraging their safe, rational and more effective (including cost-effective) use;
- to promote understanding, education and clinical training in pharmacovigilance and its effective communication to health professionals and the public".

In order to detect and assess ADRs, pharmacovigilance is based on the collection of information about the therapeutic use of medicines after marketing authorisation; most pharmacovigilance systems rely on the spontaneous reporting of adverse effects (Pal et al. 2013). The most important source of ADR information is collected through individual case safety reports (ICSRs).

The importance of pharmacovigilance for public health legislation is illustrated by the expansion of the Programme for International Drug Monitoring by the WHO. This programme began in 1968 with 10 partner countries and has continued to expand; more than 100 countries have joined the programme as of 2016. The WHO maintains a global database including information about which countries have submitted over 10 million ICSRs chronicling adverse reactions.

The Role of Healthcare Professionals

So that pharmacovigilance can be effective, all suspected ADRs must be reported in an accurate and timely manner (Alvarez-Requejo et al. 1998). In general, pharmacovigilance requires the close collaboration of various actors, such as politicians, policy officials, health administrators, the pharmaceutical industry, healthcare professionals and increasingly the general public. However, healthcare professionals have a key role in pharmacovigilance and ADR reporting in particular.

According to the WHO, healthcare professionals "maintain health in humans through the application of the principles and procedures of evidence-based medicine and caring" (WHO Education Guidelines 2016). In line with the WHO's definition, we are including the following groups under the general heading of healthcare professionals:

- Medical doctors (including general and specialised practitioners)
- Nursing professionals
- Midwifery professionals
- Dentists
- Pharmacists

However, these groups include further sub-groups and some variation also exists in the national terminology, which is reflected in the respective country chapters (see Chapter 5); healthcare professionals can be referred to as doctors, physicians, clinicians and practitioners. These terms are often country-specific and reflect the national variety of healthcare systems.

Causality Assessment and Signal Detection

With the increase of ADR reporting, establishing a causal relationship between the administration of a drug and adverse effects has become more challenging (Naidu 2013). Whereas causality assessments used to rely solely on expert judgment, automatic data processing through algorithms has become more important for determining the likelihood of a causal link. Thus, establishing a causal link between the prescription of a drug and observed effects is far from straightforward.

Causality assessment describes the systematic appraisal of reported adverse reactions in an attempt to establish a causal link between a prescribed drug and the adverse reaction.

A signal is defined as reported information about a possible causal link between a drug and the adverse effect, and signal detection is an essential element of pharmacovigilance with the goal of identifying unexpected ADRs and to inform authorities about possible regulatory actions that should be taken (Inácio et al. 2015; Kumar and Khan 2015). In order to create signals, however, more than one ICSR is needed, and the strength of the signal depends on the quantity and quality of the information. In order to detect signals, pharmacovigilance relies on databases and statistical methods to collect information with a view to establish causality between a drug and adverse reactions.

2.2   Importance of Pharmacovigilance for Biologicals

Due to the use of living cells, biologicals pose a specific challenge to pharmacovigilance. Accurate reporting of ADRs regarding the use of biologicals is especially challenging because of the restrictions in clinical trials, sensitivity to changes in the manufacturing process, the reporting of batch numbers and the establishment of valid causality assessments.

First, biologicals have distinctive features that can cause ADRs and might not be detectable in conventional clinical trials (Calvo and Zuñiga 2014). For biologicals, data from clinical trials are quite limited due to various factors, including their sample size and duration. Conditions during clinical trials differ significantly from conditions encountered under normal clinical practices. Moreover, biologicals are often prescribed only for rare diseases. In these cases, it is difficult to include a sufficient number of patients or special patient groups (such as children, the elderly or pregnant women) and to examine drug interaction in the clinical trials preceding authorisation (Giezen and Straus 2012).

Hence, it is unlikely that every risk can be identified before the drug receives market authorisation and can be administered to a large group of patients. Accordingly, it is crucial that regulatory action does not end after market approval but that the benefit-risk assessment remains an ongoing activity, ideally spanning a drug's full life cycle (Eichler et al. 2008). However, this is only possible when any adverse reaction or event of a biological is accurately reported to the competent authorities and can be traced back to the respective manufacturer.

Second, biologicals differ from small-molecule medicines in their highly complex structures and sensitivity to changes (Klein et al. 2016). Biologicals are developed in long and complex production processes involving different manufacturers and even minor changes in any step of the manufacturing process can affect the product quality and safety, e.g. through alterations of the molecular structure or non-adherence to quality standards. Potential changes in product quality and the safety profile can affect not only different products containing the same active substance, but also batches within the same medicinal product (batch-to-batch). Thus, changes, intended or unintended, could result in previously unobserved, severe ADRs, with unpredictable consequences for the consumer (Klein et al. 2016).

Third, because ADRs of biologicals can be batch-specific, it is crucial that not only the brand name, but also the batch number is accurately reported to ensure the correct and timely identification and facilitate the traceability up to the batch level (Vermeer et al. 2013). Recent studies have shown that brand-name identification is well established but that batch numbers are (still) under-reported (Klein et al. 2016).

Fourth, a drug can only be withdrawn from the market for safety reasons when a valid causality assessment is established. Yet to define this period – or the at-risk window – is especially challenging when it comes to biologicals (Giezen and Straus 2012; Arnaiz et al. 2001). Thus, calculating the risk-benefit balance and therefore deciding to withdraw a certain drug from the market is only possible with sufficiently valid data through accurate ADR reporting.

In order to ensure the correct and timely attribution of adverse events to the correct product and batch, the availability of information, such as the international non-proprietary name, the brand name, the company's name and the batch number, is necessary (Calvo and Zuñiga 2013:18).

For these reasons, timely and accurate reporting of ADRs is particularly important when it comes to the use of biologicals. Under-reporting reduces sensitivity because it underestimates the frequency and thus the impact of the problem and makes the system more vulnerable to selective reporting which may introduce a serious bias (Alvarez-Requejo et al. 1998). Adequate availability of exposure information is necessary to timely link an emerging product safety issue to the correct product and batch (Klein et al. 2016). Even though the level of evidence of case reports is often poor, spontaneous reports contribute to the majority of safety withdrawals. And when there are no doubts about the causal relationship between an adverse event and a drug, spontaneous reports may be the sole source for regulatory action (Ebbers et al. 2011).

References

Belton, K. J. and the European Pharmacovigilance Group (1997). *Attitude Survey of Adverse Drug-Reaction Reporting by Health Care Professionals across the European Union*. European Journal of Pharmacology 52: 423-427.

Alvarez-Requejo, A., Carvajal, A., Bégaud, B., Moride, Y., Vega, T., Martín Arias, L.H. (1998). *Under-Reporting of Adverse Drug Reactions: Estimate Based on a Spontaneous Reporting Scheme and a Sentinel System*. European Journal of Clinical Pharmacology 54: 483-488.

Arnaiz, J. A., Carné, X., Riba, N., Codina, C., Ribas, J., Trilla, A. (2001). *The Use of Evidence in Pharmacovigilance – Case Reports as the Reference Source for Drug Withdrawals*. European Journal of Clinical Pharmacology 57: 89-91.

Calvo, B., Zuñiga, L. (2014). *EU's New Pharmacovigilance Legislation: Considerations for Biosimilars*. Drug Safety 37: 9-18.

Ebbers, H. C., Mantel-Teeuwisse, A. K., Moors, E. H. M., Schellekens, H., Leufkens, H. C. (2011). *Today's Challenges in Pharmacovigilance: What Can We Learn from Epoetins?* Drug Safety 34(4): 273-287.

Eichler, H. G., Pignatti, F., Flamion, B., Leufkens, H., Breckenrige, A. (2008). *Balancing Early Market Access to New Drugs with the Need for Benefit/Risk Data: A Mounting Dilemma*. Nature Reviews Drug Discovery 7: 818-826.

Giezen, T. J., Straus, S. M. J. M. (2012). *Pharmacovigilance of Biosimilars: Challenges and Possible Solutions*. Generics and Biosimilars Initiative Journal 1 (3-4): 118-119.

Inácio, P., Airaksinen, M., Cavaco, A. (2015). *Language Does Not Come "in Boxes": Assessing Discrepancies between Adverse Drug Reactions Spontaneous Reporting and MedDRA® Codes in European Portuguese*. Research in Social and Administrative Pharmacy 11: 664-674.

Johnson, C.L., Hutchinson, J. A. (2015). *Pharmacovigilance in Europe*. Transplantation 99(8): 1542-1543.

Klein, K., Scholl, J. H. G., Vermeer, N. S., Broekmans, A. W., Van Puijenbroek, E. P., De Bruin, M. L., Stolk, P. (2016). *Traceability of Biologics in The Netherlands: An Analysis of Information-Recording Systems in Clinical Practice and Spontaneous ADR Reports*. Drug Safety 39: 185-192.

Kumar, A., Khan, H. (2015). *Signal Detection and Their Assessment. In Pharmacovigilance.* Open Pharmaceutical Science Journal 3: 66-73.

Pal, S. N., Duncombe, C., Falzon, D., Olsson, S. (2013). *WHO Strategy for Collecting Safety Data in Public Health Programmes: Complementing Spontaneous Reporting Systems.* Drug Safety 36: 75-81

Vermeer, N. S., Straus, S. M. J. M., Mantel-Teeuwisse, A. K., Domergue, F., Egberts, T. C. G., Leufkens, H. G. M., De Bruin, M. L. (2013). *Traceability of Biopharmaceuticals in Spontaneous Reporting Systems: A Cross-Sectional Study in the FDA Adverse Event Reporting System (FAERS) and EudraVigilance Databases.* Drug Safety 36: 617-625.

WHO (2004). *Pharmacovigilance: Ensuring the Safe Use of Medicines.* WHO Policy Perspectives on Medicines 9.

WHO (2016). *WHO Education Guidelines.* Last accessed 26.11.2016: http://whoeducationguidelines.org/content/1-definition-and-list-health-professionals

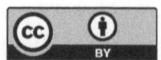

The EU Pharmacovigilance System 3

This chapter introduces pharmacovigilance in the European Union (EU); due to the multi-level nature of the EU, pharmacovigilance is described both at the European and the national level. Both levels are linked through multiple inter-institutional relations and, in combination, the European and national levels make up the EU's pharmacovigilance system.

A simplified visual representation of the system is shown in Fig. 3.1, illustrating the main connections of the most important players of the system discussed in this chapter. Depending on the regulatory procedure and the life cycle of the medicine, these actors are connected in varying networks.

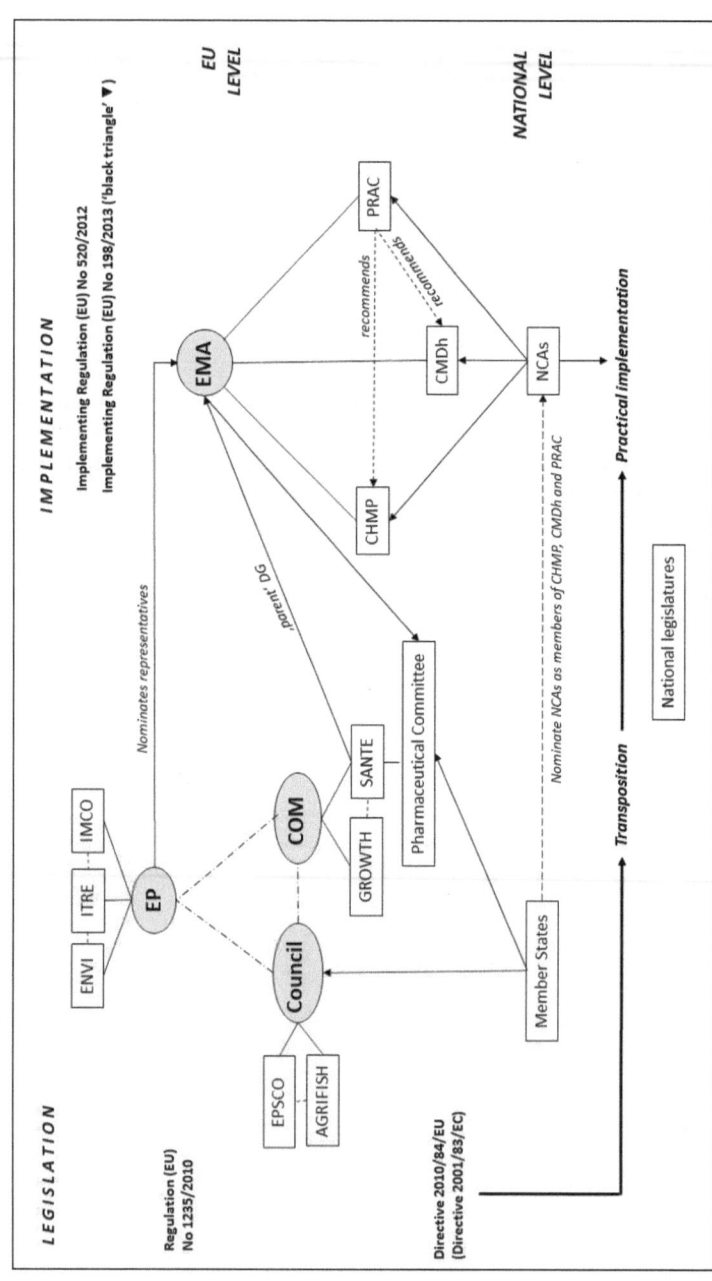

Fig. 3.1   The pharmacovigilance network on the European level

Abbreviations

- **EP**   **European Parliament**
  - ENVI   Environment, Public Health and Food Safety
  - ITRE   Industry, Research and Energy
  - IMCO   Internal Market and Consumer Protection

- **Council**
  - EPSCO   Employment, Social Policy, Health and Consumer Affairs
  - AGRIFISH   Agriculture and Fisheries

- **COM**   **European Commission**
  - SANTE   DG Health and Food Safety ('parent' DG)
  - GROWTH   DG Internal Market, Industry, Entrepreneurship and SMEs

- **EMA**   **European Medicines Agency**
  - CMHP   Committee for Medicinal Products for Human Use
  - PRAC   Pharmacovigilance Risk Assessment Committee
  - CMDh   Co-ordination Group for Mutual Recognition and Decentralised procedures – Human

- **NCAs**   **National Competent Authorities**

Direct link (e.g. through representation or supervision)

Indirect link

Organisational connection (i.e. committee or working group)

Informal connection

Legislative 'triangle' involving Council, EP and Commission

Policy making process

Recommendations

In the past, EU pharmaceuticals regulation only included the efficient authorisation of medicinal products. The regulation continues to serves a dual objective, namely the free movement of medicinal products in the EU and the protection of public health. Marketing authorisation can be obtained through a decentralised procedure by Member States or in a centralised procedure by the European Medicines Agency (EMA).[3] During the course of these procedures, medicinal products undergo risk assessment to test their quality, safety and efficacy. Thus, the assessment of risks and benefits before marketing is the cornerstone of authorisation.

Hence, the emphasis was traditionally put on the risk assessment before marketing, and the continuous assessment of authorised products used to be neglected (see Abraham and Lewis 2000). In the 1990s, this began to change when the EU passed a series of legislations dedicated to pharmacovigilance. Today, EU regulation covers the whole life cycle of medicinal products: drug development and manufacturing, clinical trials, marketing authorisation and pharmacovigilance (see Scholz 2015). This includes not only the spontaneous reporting of adverse drug reactions (ADRs), but also systematic reporting through risk management plans (Moore and Begaud 2010).

In this chapter, we give an overview of the pharmacovigilance system in the EU. First, we introduce the main legislative and executive institutions in the EU, namely the European Commission (Commission), the Council of Ministers (Council) and the European Parliament (EP) as well as the actors responsible for implementing pharmacovigilance policy. We then give a brief overview of pharmacovigilance legislative developments, notably Directive 2001/83/EC and the subsequent reform through Directive 2010/84/EU and conclude by presenting the most important changes brought about by the reform Directive and discussing the ADR provisions in the Directive.

---

3   Pharmaceuticals authorised through the centralised procedure can be marketed throughout the entire EU. For some medicinal products, such as those derived from biotechnology processes, the centralised procedure is mandatory. For medicinal products outside of the scope of the centralised procedure, pharmaceutical companies can opt for decentralised procedures, whereby these products can then only be marketed in a few Member States.

3.1   EU Institutions and Pharmacovigilance Actors

For a better understanding of the EU system of pharmacovigilance, it is important to distinguish between two sets of actors. The first set of actors comprises the EU institutions which pass pharmaceutical regulations and set the policy framework for pharmacovigilance. The Commission, the Council and the EP are the institutions with legislative and executive tasks in the EU. Together, they can be conceived of as a legislative triangle.

The European Commission performs a variety of functions and is the institution which is supposed to represent European interests. Varying policy issues are dealt with by so-called Directorate Generals (DGs); DG Health and Food Safety (SANTE) handles the pharmaceuticals regulation. DG SANTE is also the "parent" DG of EMA, which means that representatives of this DG are important points of reference for the day-to-day activities of the agency. However, representatives of both DGs are members of the EMA Management Board which is the main steering body of the agency. Among its many functions, the initiation of legislation is a key task of the Commission. In addition, EU legislation can only be adopted based on proposals by the Commission. Regarding its executive functions, the Commission is supported by an expert group, the Pharmaceutical Committee, which was established in 1975; this committee consists of representatives of the Member States and EMA. Its main tasks relate to the implementation of pharmaceuticals legislation and particularly Directive 2001/83/EC, and it is supervised by DG SANTE.

The Council of Ministers has primarily legislative functions and is the institution which represents the Member States. Depending on the policy subject at stake, the Council convenes and negotiates in varying configurations with different national ministers present at meetings. Regarding the revision of Directive 2001/83/EC, the Council convened in two different configurations: the Employment, Social Policy, Health and Consumer Affairs (EPSCO) group as well as Agriculture and Fisheries (AGRIFISH). Together with the EP, the Council passes legislative acts such as the aforementioned pharmacovigilance legislation.

The European Parliament (EP) representing the people of Europe is, together with the Council, the legislature of the EU. Legislative proposals initiated by the Commission are dealt with by one or more parliamentary committees. Directive 2001/83/EC, for instance, was handled by the Environment, Public Health and Food Safety (ENVI) committee with two other committees providing further opinions on the legislative proposal.[4] The EP is entitled to send two representatives to the

---

4   Internal Market and Consumer Protection (IMCO) and Industry, Research and Energy (ITRE).

EMA Management Board. Usually, scientific experts are sent to represent the EP. As part of the legislature, the EP also plays an important role regarding budgetary oversight and control of EMA. However, the EP plays a limited role regarding the practical implementation of pharmacovigilance policies.

The second set of actors is responsible for implementing pharmacovigilance policy at the EU and national levels, based on the legislation passed by the EU institutions. As will be explained in Chapter 4, national legislatures have to transpose EU directives into national law. In addition, implementing legislation is adopted by the EU at the EU level. Yet this set also comprises the EMA, the national competent authorities, and pharmaceutical companies and other stakeholders.

The main task of the <u>European Medicines Agency</u> (EMA) is to coordinate the evaluation of medicinal products and to advise the EU institutions and the Member States on any issue relating to pharmaceuticals regulation. Since it began operating in 1995, the agency has become a central actor regarding various aspects of pharmaceuticals regulation and has a crucial role in providing the infrastructure for EU pharmacovigilance. For its scientific assessments, the agency relies on a number of committees, including the Committee for Medicinal Products for Human Use (CMPH), which issues recommendations to the Commission regarding the centralised authorisation procedure. In addition, since 2012, the Pharmacovigilance Risk Assessment Committee (PRAC) assesses and monitors the safety of medicinal products. PRAC issues opinions and recommendations about centralised and decentralised authorisation procedures.

The EMA's <u>EudraVigilance database</u> is an internet-based information system where reports of suspected adverse reactions are collected. It is legally required that ADRs occurring in the EU must be included in the database by the Member States and marketing authorisation holders.

Furthermore, the pharmacovigilance system of the EU relies heavily on the <u>Member States and their national competent authorities</u>. As can be seen in Fig. 3.1, Member State actors are involved in almost all pharmacovigilance activities. Drawing on national expertise and resources, the national competent authorities are at the centre of pharmacovigilance implementation and enforcement activities (see European Commission 2016a). These authorities are not only at the centre of practical implementation at the national level, but also represented at the EU level in the various EMA committees dealing with authorisation and pharmacovigilance.

At the EU level, the Co-ordination Group for Mutual Recognition and De-centralised Procedures (CMDh) is in charge of decision-making when medicinal products are marketed through the decentralised procedure. In addition, the Strengthening Collaboration for Operating Pharmacovigilance in Europe (SCOPE) Joint Action initiative supports the operation of EU pharmacovigilance by delivering training, tools and templates to support best practices (European Commission 2015). The European Network of Centres for Pharmacoepidemiology and Pharmacovigilance (ENCePP) also aims to improve the science and practice of pharmacovigilance.

At the national level, the national competent authorities are the central bodies supervising the collection of information about suspected ADRs submitted by healthcare professionals, marketing authorisation holders and patients. By doing so, these authorities provide for resources, knowledge and expertise regarding causality assessment and signal detection (European Commission 2016b).

Pharmacovigilance is based on the EMA's close connections with the pharmaceutical industry (see Wiktorwowicz et al. 2012) and include risk management plans and post-authorisation safety studies which are important elements of the authorisation procedure and product surveillance after marketing. Regarding pharmacovigilance, marketing authorisation holders have to comply with a number of stipulations laid down in EU legislation. For instance, they have to appoint a responsible person in charge of pharmacovigilance who serves as the main contact point for regulatory authorities. In addition, marketing authorisation holders are also legally obligated to report ADRs.

Finally, some additional stakeholders are significant in the proper implementation of the EU pharmacovigilance legislation.

Regulation (EC) No 726/2004 explicitly mentions the participation of stakeholders in EU pharmaceuticals regulation. In the framework of EMA, a network of European patient and consumer organisations as well as a Patients' and Consumers' Working Party have been established.

The reform of the pharmacovigilance system by Directive 2010/84/EU has introduced the possibility for patients to report suspected side effects directly, either to the national competent authorities or the marketing authorisation holders. As explained below, the Directive also aims to simplify and facilitate individual reporting by patients.

3.2   Legislative Developments

Although pharmaceuticals regulation in the EU dates back to the 1960s, pharmacovigilance was neglected until the 1990s, when the EU began to pass a series of legislations dedicated to pharmacovigilance (see Abraham and Lewis 2000). Already, Directive 93/39/EEC stated that Member States must establish pharmacovigilance systems and encourage healthcare professionals to report ADRs. Marketing authorisation holders were also requested to appoint a qualified person responsible for pharmacovigilance.

At that time, EU pharmaceuticals regulation consisted of various pieces of legislation that were interconnected in complex ways. Hence, with a view to simplification, the various pieces were codified in a single text, leading to Directive 2001/83/EC. This Directive is the legal basis of the EU legislation on pharmacovigilance and has been amended 10 times. Compared with Directive 93/39/EEC, the requirements for Member States and marketing authorisation holders to set up and maintain pharmacovigilance systems did not change substantially. Hence, the relevant provisions, introduced in essence in the early 1990s, were merely consolidated in Title IX of Directive 2001/83/EC which was dedicated to pharmacovigilance.

In 2006, the Commission initiated a public consultation with a view to reform the pharmacovigilance system. The goals stated by the Commission included clarifying stakeholder responsibility, ensuring the involvement of varying stakeholders (including healthcare professionals and stakeholders), and clarifying duplications and responsibilities. The public consultation was accompanied by an assessment report, which found "disparities and inconsistencies resulting from a non-optimal compliance of both national law and practice with the EC regulations" (European Commission 2006).

Based on the consultation, the Commission issued a legislative proposal in December 2008. In this proposal, the Commission explained that it was aiming at the following objectives: better protection of public health, proper internal market functioning, and a simplification of the current rules and procedures (European Commission 2008).

The proposal was then discussed by the Member States in the respective Council working group throughout the next year. After beginning preparatory talks in late 2009, the Council and the EP engaged in a series of informal meetings (so-called trialogues) with a view to ensuring the quick adoption of the Directive (Council of the European Union 2010). In September 2010, the EP passed Directive 2010/84/EU with a majority, thus concluding the legislative procedure.

Additional legislation is important to maintain the EU pharmacovigilance system. While Directive 2010/84/EU covers pharmacovigilance regarding decentralised authorisation, Regulation (EU) No 1235/2010 covers the centralised authorisation procedure. Operational aspects for these legislations were adopted through Commission Implementing Regulation No 520/2012. For instance, the regulation stipulates that individual case safety reports concerning biologicals must contain the batch numbers. Furthermore, Implementing Regulation No 198/2013 introduces the "black triangle" (▼). The recital of the Regulation is as follows:

Some medicinal products for human use are subject to additional monitoring because of their specific safety profile, including medicinal products with a new active substance, biological medicinal products and products for which post-authorisation data are required (see also James 2014). As the Commission explains on its website, the black triangle (▼) aims to highlight to patients the importance of reporting suspected side effects stemming from the medicines they are taking, improving their safety.

A product which is subject to additional monitoring is included in an online up-to-date list which is publicly available on the EMA homepage. All products on this list must display an inverted black triangle symbol (▼) and include a standardised explanatory sentence in both their summary of product characteristics and in the package leaflet (European Commission 2014: 15). This additional list was launched by the EMA in April 2013 and draws attention to and increases transparency for patients in order to encourage the reporting of suspected adverse effects.

Finally, Regulation (EU) No 1027/2012 and Directive 2012/26/EU amended the legislation due to the withdrawal of a medicine called Mediator (benfluorex) (cf. Box 5.4 in Chapter 5.4). These amendments require a marketing authorisation holder to notify the competent authority of that Member State when a medicine is withdrawn from the market.

Complementing legislation, the EU system of pharmacovigilance comprises a set of technical principles described in respective guidance documents. These principles ensure that the requirements of pharmaceuticals regulation are applied in a uniform manner. These principles include good manufacturing practice (GMP), good distribution practice (GDP) and good pharmacovigilance practice (GVP). The GVP guidance documents aim to facilitate pharmacovigilance in the EU and cover medicines authorised through both the centralised and the decentralised procedure.

3.3   The Pharmacovigilance Reform: Directive 2010/84/EU and Article 102

The aim of the new pharmacovigilance Directive 2010/84/EU is "to improve the operation of Union law on the pharmacovigilance of medicinal products" (Recital 3). In summary, the new legislation brought about the following changes to the EU system of pharmacovigilance:

- Extension of the scope for additional monitoring (e.g. of biologicals)
- Competent authorities may require additional monitoring for products that are subject to studies after marketing
- Medicinal products subject to additional monitoring are required to be identified by the black triangle (▼) and to be included in a publicly available list
- Patients are encouraged to report ADRs directly to the competent authorities
- ADRs are extended to include medication errors and overdose

The reform of the EU pharmacovigilance system aimed at facilitating ADR reporting with a specific emphasis on the identification of biologicals (European Commission 2007). To this end, the Commission enhanced Articles 101 and 102 which laid down provisions in this respect (Box 3.1). In these articles, three elements can be identified: 1) Member States must take measures to encourage healthcare professionals to report ADRs; 2) Member States may impose specific requirements to do so; 3) Member States must establish a pharmacovigilance system. The revision of these provisions through Directive 2010/84/EU mainly extends the latter element, whereas the former two elements were retained as described.

The extension of these provisions proved to be a controversial subject with Member States. Based on the initial provision of the Commission proposal, Article 102 alone sparked 14 comments, with nine Member States requesting changes (Council of European Union 2009). Throughout the legislative procedure, the exact wording of these provisions was subject to much discussion among Member States.

In total, the parliamentary committees dealing with the Commission proposal tabled more than 70 amendments. Throughout the informal trialogue meetings with the Council, a compromise text was developed which did not retain all amendments in the proposed wording, but which maintained key stipulations included by the EP.

Pharmacovigilance provisions in Article 102 of Directive 2010/84/EU were adopted as follows (Box 3.1):

The Member States shall:

a. take all appropriate measures to encourage patients, doctors, pharmacists and other healthcare professionals to report suspected adverse reactions to the national competent authority; for these tasks, organisations representing consumers, patients and healthcare professionals may be involved as appropriate;

In the Commission proposal and in the Council discussions, patients were not originally included. The inclusion of patients in this stipulation is due to the amendment of the EP which was eventually retained in the compromise text; in the literature, there is no agreement on whether patients' inclusion improves pharmacovigilance by extending the scope of actors reporting ADRs or whether such inclusion leads to information overload and a diminution of the quality of the reports (see e.g. de Langen et al. 2008). The inclusion of consumer and patients' organisations is also due to the parliamentary amendment; their role, however, was diminished in the compromise text.

b. facilitate patient reporting through the provision of alternative reporting formats in addition to web-based formats;

In connection with the general inclusion of patients in ADR reporting in point a), this stipulation was also included due to parliamentary amendment.

c. take all appropriate measures to obtain accurate and verifiable data for the scientific evaluation of suspected adverse reaction reports;

d. ensure that the public is given important information on pharmacovigilance concerns relating to the use of a medicinal product in a timely manner through publication on the web portal and through other means of publicly available information as necessary;

The wording of point c) was subject to much discussion among Member States. In contrast to the original stipulation of the Commission proposal, the Council added the provision relating pharmacovigilance to scientific evaluation. This was absent in the proposal which only spoke of "high quality information". A parliamentary amendment extending this "quality" stipulation to not only reports but also databases was not included in the compromise text. However, the stipulation on risk communication due to ADR reporting in point d) was included by the EP and retained in the final text.

e. ensure, through the methods for collecting information and where necessary through the follow-up of suspected adverse reaction reports, that all appropriate measures are taken to identify clearly any biological medicinal product prescribed, dispensed, or sold in their territory which is the subject of a suspected adverse reaction report, with due regard to the name of the medicinal product, in accordance with Article 1(20), and the batch number;

Based on the Commission proposal, the exact wording regarding the identification of biologicals was also the subject of much discussion among the Member States.

However, a substantial amendment was made by the EP. First, the EP extended the scope of the stipulation to suspected adverse reaction reports. Second, in contrast to the original stipulation, the EP explicitly included the name of the medicinal product, the international non-proprietary name, the name of the marketing authorisation holder and the batch number. The members of the respective committee justified the amendment with the concern that the Commission proposal lacked details on how to identify biologicals. According to this view, a lack of details would lead to different national pharmacovigilance approaches for medicinal products subject to centralised authorisation. In the compromise text, the elements of reporting, including the batch number, were maintained. In addition, the wording of the stipulation was softened and the references to EudraVigilance and standard reporting formats were deleted.

f. take the necessary measures to ensure that a marketing authorisation holder who fails to discharge the obligations laid down in this Title is subject to effective, proportionate and dissuasive penalties.

For the purposes of point (a) and (e) of the first paragraph the Member States may impose specific obligations on doctors, pharmacists and other healthcare professionals.

In the original stipulation of the Commission proposal and the various versions of the Council discussions, the imposition of specific obligations were only foreseen for point (a), hence the general reporting requirements. In its amendment, the EP extended the possibility of imposing obligations to point (e), hence the reporting details regarding biologicals. The Commission also included the following stipulation: "Reporting of suspected adverse reactions due to medication errors should be on a 'no blame' basis, and should be legally privileged" (European Parliament 2010).[5]

Relating to the justification regarding the specific elements of reporting in point (e), the EP reasoned that this amendment would not only increase the clarity of the provision, but would also strengthen the legal basis for requesting from health professionals requirements regarding the identification of biologicals. While the extension of specific obligations to point (e) was retained, the latter amendment was not included in the compromise text.

---

5 During the parliamentary committee discussions, an additional amendment was proposed whereupon medication errors could have been reported anonymously. However, this amendment was not included by the responsible rapporteur in the EP report on amendments.

Tab. 3.1 Development of Article 102 of Directive 2010/84/EU

Commission proposal 12/2008	Council 03/2010	Council 04/2010	EP amendments 06/2010	Council 06/2010
The Member States shall:				
(1) take all appropriate measures to encourage doctors, pharmacists and other healthcare professionals to report suspected adverse reactions to the national competent authority or the marketing authorisation holder;	(1) take all appropriate measures to encourage doctors, pharmacists and other healthcare professionals to report suspected adverse reactions to the national competent authority or the marketing authorisation holder;	(1) take all appropriate measures to encourage doctors, pharmacists and other healthcare professionals to report suspected adverse reactions to the national competent authority or the marketing authorisation holder;	(1) take all appropriate measures to encourage patients, doctors, pharmacists and other healthcare professionals to report suspected adverse reactions to the national competent authority; or the marketing authorisation holder; these measures shall include training for health professionals and a public information campaign for patients. Patients' and consumer organisations shall be involved in providing information to patients and in developing public information campaigns in cooperation with regulatory bodies.	(1) take all appropriate measures to encourage patients, doctors, pharmacists and other healthcare professionals to report suspected adverse reactions to the national competent authority or the marketing authorisation holder; for these tasks, consumer organisations, patients organisations and healthcare professionals organisations scientific societies may be involved as appropriate.
			(1a) facilitate direct patient reporting through the provision of alternative reporting formats in addition to web-based formats;	(1a) facilitate patient reporting through the provision of alternative reporting formats in addition to web-based formats;

Commission proposal 12/2008	Council 03/2010	Council 04/2010	EP amendments 06/2010	Council 06/2010
(2) ensure that adverse reaction reports contain the highest-quality information possible;	(2) ensure that all appropriate measures are taken to obtain accurate and verifiable data for the scientific evaluation of adverse reaction reports and that they contain the highest-quality information possible	(2) ensure that all appropriate measures are taken to obtain accurate and verifiable data for the scientific evaluation of adverse reaction reports and that they contain the highest-quality information possible	(2) ensure that adverse reaction reports *and databases* contain the highest-quality information possible; *(2a) ensure that the public is given important information in good time on pharmacovigilance concerns relating to the use of a medicinal product through publication on the web portal and through other means of public information as necessary;*	(2) ensure that all appropriate measures are taken to obtain accurate and verifiable data for the scientific evaluation of suspected adverse reaction reports and that they contain the highest-quality information possible; (2a) ensure that the public is given important information in good time on pharmacovigilance concerns relating to the use of a medicinal product through publication on the web portal and through other means of public information as necessary;

Commission proposal 12/2008	Council 03/2010	Council 04/2010	EP amendments 06/2010	Council 06/2010
(3) through the methods of collecting information and where necessary through the follow-up of adverse reaction reports, ensure that any biological medicinal product prescribed, dispensed or sold in their territory which is the subject of an adverse reaction report is identifiable;	(3) through the methods of collecting information and where necessary through the follow-up of adverse reaction reports, ensure that any biological medicinal product prescribed, dispensed or sold in their territory which is the subject of an adverse reaction report is identifiable;	(3) make sure, through the methods of collecting information and where necessary through the follow-up of adverse reaction reports, ensure that all appropriate measures are taken to identify any biological medicinal product prescribed, dispensed or sold in their territory which is the subject of an adverse reaction report is identifiable;	(3) ensure that any biological medicinal product prescribed, dispensed or sold in their territory which is the subject of *a report on a suspected* adverse reaction is identifiable *by, where available, the name of the MAH, the INN, the name of the medicinal product and the batch number, using the standard forms and procedures developed in accordance with Article 25(1) of the Regulation (EC) No 726/2004 and taking due account of the developments within the EudraVigilance system.*[1]	(3) make sure, through the methods of collecting information and where necessary through the follow-up of suspected adverse reaction reports, ensure that all appropriate measures are taken to identify any biological medicinal product prescribed, dispensed or sold in their territory which is the subject of an suspected adverse reaction report is identifiable; with due regard to the name of the medicinal product (in accordance with Article 1(20)) and the batch number.
(4) take the necessary measures to ensure that a marketing authorisation holder who fails to discharge the obligations laid down in this Title is subject to effective, proportionate and dissuasive penalties.	(4) take the necessary measures to ensure that a marketing authorisation holder who fails to discharge the obligations laid down in this Title is subject to effective, proportionate and dissuasive penalties.	(4) take the necessary measures to ensure that a marketing authorisation holder who fails to discharge the obligations laid down in this Title is subject to effective, proportionate and dissuasive penalties.	(4) take the necessary measures to ensure that a marketing authorisation holder who fails to discharge the obligations laid down in this Title is subject to effective, proportionate and dissuasive penalties.	(4) take the necessary measures to ensure that a marketing authorisation holder who fails to discharge the obligations laid down in this Title is subject to effective, proportionate and dissuasive penalties.

Commission proposal 12/2008	Council 03/2010	Council 04/2010	EP amendments 06/2010	Council 06/2010
For the purposes of point (1) of the first paragraph the Member States may impose specific requirements on doctors, pharmacists and other healthcare professionals respecting the reporting of suspected serious or unexpected adverse reactions.	For the purposes of point (1) of the first paragraph the Member States may impose specific requirements on doctors, pharmacists and other health-care professionals respecting the reporting of suspected serious or unexpected adverse reactions.	For the purposes of point (1) of the first paragraph the Member States may impose specific requirements on doctors, pharmacists and other healthcare professionals respecting the reporting of suspected serious or unexpected adverse reactions.	For the purposes of *points (1) and (3)* of the first paragraph the Member States may impose specific requirements on doctors, pharmacists and other healthcare professionals. *Reporting of suspected adverse reactions due to medication errors should be on a 'no blame' basis, and should be legally privileged* [not to be used in court proceedings].	For the purposes of point (1) and (3) of the first paragraph the Member States may impose specific requirements on doctors, pharmacists and other health-care professionals respecting the reporting of suspected serious or unexpected adverse reactions.

[1] Justification: The present proposal lacks details about how to clearly identify biological medicinal products and creates the risk of 27 different approaches (…) providing a number of identifiers for biologicals and is linked to an amendment to Article 25 of the Regulation (EC) No 726/2004, which assigns to the European Medicines Agency (EMA) the task of developing forms for adverse event reporting for biological medicinal products (…) ensure that a legal basis is created to request from healthcare professionals and pharmacists requirements relating specifically to the identification of biologics.

References

Abraham, J., Lewis, G. (2000). *Regulating Medicines in Europe – Competition, Expertise and Public Health.* Routledge: London and New York.

Council of the European Union (2009). Note from General Secretariat of the Council to Working Party on Pharmaceuticals and Medical Devices, 7996/1/09, Brussels, 4 May 2009.

Council of the European Union (2010). Note from General Secretariat of the Council to Working Party on Pharmaceuticals and Medical Devices, 9697/3/10, Brussels, 17 June 2010.

De Langen, J., Van Hunsel, F., Passier, A., De Jong-Van Den Berg, L., Van Grootheest, K. (2008). Adverse Drug Reaction Reporting by Patients in The Netherlands. Three Years of Experience. Drug Safety, 31 (6): 515-524.

European Commission (2006). *Commission Public Consultation: An Assessment of the Community System of Pharmacovigilance.* 15.03.2006.

European Commission (2007). *Strategy to Better Protect Public Health by Strengthening and Rationalizing EU Pharmacovigilance.* Public Consultation on Legislative Proposals. Brussels, 05.12.2007.

European Commission (2008). *Proposal for a Directive of the European Parliament and of the Council Amending, as Regards Pharmacovigilance, Directive 2001/83/EC on the Community Code Relating to Medicinal Products for Human Use.* COM(2008) 665 final, Brussels, 10.12.2008.

European Commission (2014). *Summary Record.* Pharmaceutical Committee, 26 March 2014, PHARM 659.

European Commission (2015). *Overview of Member States' Biennial Reports on Audits of their Pharmacovigilance Systems (2013 Reporting Year).* Pharmaceutical Committee, 21 October 2015, PHARM 693.

European Commission (2016a). *Pharmacovigilance Related Activities of Member States and the European Medicines Agency Concerning Medicinal Products for Human Use (2012-2014).* COM(2016) 498 final, Brussels, 08.08.2016.

European Commission (2016b). *Commission Staff Working Document Accompanying the Document Commission Report Pharmacovigilance Related Activities of Member States and the European Medicines Agency Concerning Medicinal Products for Human Use (2012-2014).* SWD(2016) 284 final, Brussels, 08.08.2016.

European Parliament (2010). *Report on the Proposal for a Directive of the European Parliament and of the Council Amending, as Regards Pharmacovigilance, Directive 2001/83/EC on the Community Code Relating to Medicinal Products for Human Use.* (COM(2008)0665 – C6-0514/2008 – 2008/0260(COD)), A7-0159-2010, 02.06.2010.

James, C. (2014). *Adverse Drug Reaction Reporting. NHS Education for Scotland 2014.* Last accessed on 04.10.2016: http://www.nhstaysideadtc.scot.nhs.uk/netFormulary/PDF/Adverse%20drug%20reaction%20reporting.pdf.

Moore, N., Bégaud, B. (2010). *Improving Pharmacovigilance in Europe.* The BMJ 340: c1694.

Scholz, N. (2015). *Medicinal Products in the European Union. The Legal Framework for Medicines for Human Use.* European Parliamentary Research Service, April 2015-PE 554.174.

Wiktorwowicz, M., Lexchin, J., Moscou, K. (2012). *Pharmacovigilance in Europe and North America: Divergent Approaches.* Social Science and Medicine, 75: 165-170.

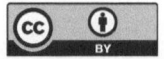

Timely and Correct Transposition of Pharmacovigilance across Member States 4

There has long been a vague supposition that the European Union (EU) has a transposition problem (Groenleer et al. 2010; Kaeding 2006, 2007a, b, 2008a, b, c, 2012; Kaeding and Versluis 2014; Klika 2015a, 2015b; Mastenbroek and Kaeding 2006, 2007; Schmälter 2017; Steunenberg et al. 2006; Steunenberg and Kaeding 2009). This chapter offers a first assessment of the timeliness of national transposition processes for all EU Member States and their respective national pharmacovigilance systems.

When the timeliness of national transposition processes of pharmacovigilance for all EU Member States is considered, this assessment shows that many countries have a serious transposition problem in their national pharmacovigilance systems.

4.1 Timely Transposition of Directive 2010/84/EU across Member States

Fig. 4.1 calculates the difference between the transposition deadline set in the EU pharmacovigilance Directive (21.07.2012) and the date of publication of the first and last national transposition instruments. The figure shows the delays in weeks for the 101 national implementing measures of Directive 2010/84/EU.

Whereas the average number of implementing measures needed to transpose the EU pharmacovigilance directive was 3.6, 12 Member States communicated only one transposing instrument. However, Malta, Hungary and Lithuania needed nine, 13 and 14 instruments, respectively.

In addition, only 16 out of the 101 (15 percent) national implementing measures were transposed on time. On the extreme end of the late transposition continuum are Finland, Spain, Poland and Slovenia; they transposed their first national implementing measures more than one year after the transposition deadline had expired.

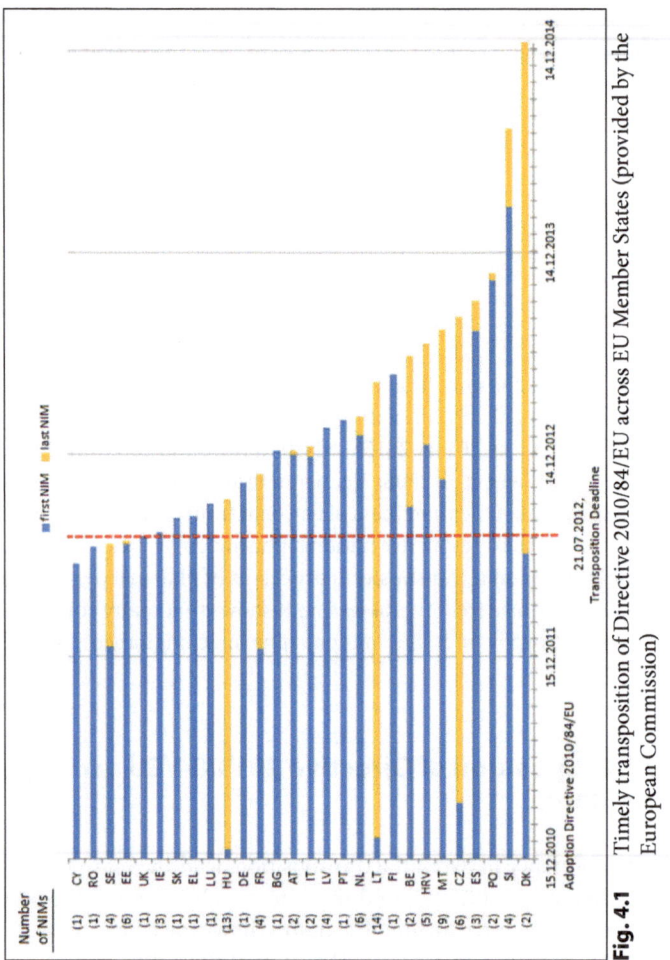

Fig. 4.1 Timely transposition of Directive 2010/84/EU across EU Member States (provided by the European Commission)

Overall, it appears that EU transposition deficits in European pharmacovigilance are not a statistical illusion. Almost 85 percent of the national transposition instruments are not transposed on time, and in fact are delayed up to more than two years.

Cross-country variance in transposing the EU pharmacovigilance Directive is significant. There is a significant difference between the laggards (Denmark and Slovenia) and the champions (Cyprus, Romania, Sweden, Estonia, the United Kingdom and Ireland).

4.2   Correct Transposition of Directive 2010/84/EU across Member States

Many Member States have endorsed so-called guiding principles for transposing EU legislation. These principles aim at policy makers and lawyers across government bodies and explain what is needed to correctly implement EU legislation.

When EU legislation is transposed, the aim should be to avoid going beyond the minimum requirements of the legal instrument being transposed. Taking such an approach will ensure that EU legislation does not create unnecessary legislative burdens. Furthermore, any gold-plating by extending the scope, adding in some way to the substantive requirement, not taking full advantage of any derogations, retaining pre-existing national standards where they are higher than those required by EU law, or implementing early before the date given in a directive, should be either avoided or eventually cleared by a reducing regulation committee. Another guiding implementation principle is to always use copy-out for transposition where it is available, except where doing so would adversely affect national interests.

In the following sections, the report analyses all national implementing measures for the six Member States (the United Kingdom, Finland, Poland, France, Portugal and Germany) under investigation. To assess whether they followed the above-mentioned guiding implementing principles, we split the analysis according to two aspects: processes and actors on the one hand, and quality and content on the other hand.

4.2.1   Correct Transposition – Processes and Actors

Table 4.1 summarises the findings of the "processes and actors" analysis and is guided by the order of the following questions:

1. What is the name, what is the type of legal instrument and who signed the national implementing measure (NIM)?
2. Was there a transposition plan, and did the actors' legal departments participate in this plan?
3. Is there a reducing regulation committee or similar, were expert groups consulted and does the NIM provide for a ministerial review?

Tab. 4.1 Correct transposition of Directive 2010/84/EU across EU Member States – processes and actors

	United Kingdom	Finland	France	Poland	Portugal	Germany
Name	UK Statutory Instrument 2012 No 1916. The Human Medicine Regulation 19/07/2012.	Laki 330/2013. Amendment to the Medicines Act.	Loi del'Etat 2011-2012. Décret 2012-1244. Arrêté du 8 novembre 2012 (R.5121-21). Arrêté du 8 novembre 2012 (R.5121-45)..	Ustawa z dnia 27 września 2013 r. o zmianie ustawy. Rozporządzenie Ministra Zdrowia z dnia 5 listopada 2013 r. zmieniające rozporządzenie w sprawie wymagań dotyczących oznakowania opakowań produktu leczniczego i treści ulotki.	Decree Law 20/2013 (14th February 2013).	Zweites Gesetz zur Änderung arznei-mittelrechtlicher und anderer Vorschriften.
Which Type?	Statutory Instrument (Regulation by Secretary of State and Minister).	Amendment to existing legislation.	Law. Presidential Decree Law. Ministerial Enactment.	Law. Ministerial Order.	Governmental Decree Law.	Law.
Who Signed?	Secretary of State; Minister for Health, Social Services and Public Safety.	President of the Republic; Minister of Social Affairs and Health.	President of the Republic; Prime Minister; Minister of Justice; Minister of Economy, Finances and Industry; Minister for Work, Employment and Health; Minister of Higher Education and Research; Prime Minister; Minister of Social Affairs and Health; Managing Director for Health (in delegation by Minister); Managing Director for Health (in delegation by Minister).	Adopted by Parliament Signed by President and the Minister of Health.	Prime Minister; Minister of Health; Approved by President.	President; Chancellor; Minister of Health.

	United Kingdom	Finland	France	Poland	Portugal	Germany
National Transposition Plan?	Impact Assessment available.	No evidence.	No evidence.	No.	No evidence.	Plan of action (*Aktionsplan 2013-2015*).
Participation of Legal Departments?	No evidence.	No evidence.	No evidence.	No evidence.	No evidence.	No evidence of participation, although the Health Ministry has its own legal department (*Justiziarrat*).
Participation of Reducing Regulation Committee?	Yes. Cooperation with the Reducing Regulation Committee.	No evidence. There is, however, the cross-ministry expert group (Better Regulation Consultative Committee).	No.	No evidence. There is, however, a Supreme Audit Office to reduce bureaucracy.	No evidence. There are, however, two programmes for legislative simplification that are currently running (*Programa Simplex / Programa Legislar Melhor*).	No evidence. There is, however, a reducing regulation committee (*Nationaler Normenkontrollrat*).
Consultation of Expert Groups?	Public consultation on implementation of Directive. More than 500 parties were contacted (Consultation MLX 374 from 06.12.2011 to 28.02.2012).	No evidence.	No evidence.	No evidence.	Consultation of healthcare professionals' associations, pharmaceutical industry associations and patients' organizations.	Consultation of 36 associations and seven experts.

4.2.2   Correct Transposition – Quality and Content

Table 4.2 summarises the findings of the "quality and content" analysis based on the following questions:

1. Has Directive 2010/84/EU been copied, or has new or existing legislation been used?
2. Is the national implementing measure longer than the original legislation?
3. Does the national implementing measure exceed the requirements of Directive 2010/84/EU?
4. Was the national implementing measure transposed before the transposition deadline on July 21st, 2012?

Tab. 4.2 Correct transposition of Directive 2010/84/EU across EU Member States – quality and content

	United Kingdom	Finland	France	Poland	Portugal	Germany
Has Directive 2010/84/EU Been Copied?	Copy-out method. Only minor changes in wording that do not affect the meaning.	No similarities with the Directive's text can be found.	No similarities with the Directive's text can be found.	No similarities with the Directive's text can be found.	Copy-out Method Only minor changes in wording that do not affect the meaning.	No similarities with the Directive's text can be found Meaning of Article 102 (e) was weakened by saying that national authorities *can impose* further measures to ensure correct identification and traceability of biological products.
New or Existing Legislation?	Adapting and replacing already existing legislation.	Adapting and replacing already existing legislation.	Adapting and replacing already existing legislation.	Adapting and replacing existing legislation.	Adapting and replacing existing legislation.	Adapting and replacing already existing legislation.
Length of NIM	53 words for transposing Article 102 (e).	Three Articles out of 17 Articles of the NIM relate to Article 102 (e).	Loi de l'Etat (25 pages, 48 Articles), Décret (16 pages), Arrêté (each one page).	Law (30 pages). Ministerial Order (three pages).	112 pages (205 articles and four annexes).	36 pages in total. Article 102 implemented in three articles, each nine sentences.
Risk of Gold-Plating?	No.	Difficult to detect because the Directive was not transposed word by word.	Difficult to detect because the Directive was not transposed word by word.	No.	No.	No.
Transposition of NIM before Deadline?	19 days before the deadline's expiration.	Delayed.	Delayed.	Delayed.	Delayed.	Delayed.

All in all, however, Member States hardly pay any attention to the above-mentioned guiding implementing principles. The EU also has a transposition problem in terms of incorrect transposition. Processes, the number of actors, the quality and the content of national implementing measures vary greatly across the selected EU Member States, leading to a great deal of diversity across Europe.

This chapter demonstrated that the transposition of EU legislation into national law remains a challenge across the EU. Yet by now, the formal transposition of Directive 2010/84/EU on pharmacovigilance has been completed in all Member States. In the following chapter, we analyse whether the transposition is also complied with in practice. With a focus on six EU Member States (the United Kingdom, Finland, Poland, France, Portugal and Germany), we depict national ADR reporting systems, examine which challenges remain, and identify best practices in order to improve existing pharmacovigilance frameworks.

References

Groenleer, M., Kaeding, M., Versluis, E. (2010). *Regulatory Governance through EU Agencies? The Role of the European Agencies for Maritime and Aviation Safety in the Implementation of European Transport Legislation.* Journal of European Public Policy 17 (8): 1212-1230.

Kaeding, M. (2006). *Determinants of Transposition Delay in the European Union.* Journal of Public Policy 26 (3): 229-253.

Kaeding, M. (2007a). *Better Regulation in the European Union – Lost in Translation or Full Steam Ahead? The Transposition of EU Transport Directives across Member States.* Leiden: Leiden University Press (224 pages).

Kaeding, M. (2007b). *Administrative Convergence Actually – An Assessment of the European Commission's Best Practices for Transposition of EU Legislation in France, Germany, Italy, Sweden and Greece.* Journal of European Integration 29 (4): 425-446.

Kaeding, M. (2008a). *In Search of Better Quality of EU Regulations for Prompt Transposition: The Brussels Perspective.* European Law Journal 14(5): 583-603.

Kaeding, M. (2008b). *Lost in Translation or Full Steam Ahead? The Transposition of EU Transport Directives across EU Member States.* European Union Politics 9 (1): 115-144.

Kaeding, M. (2008c). *In Good Times and Bad: Legal Transposition in the European Union. Necessary Conditions for Timely Transposition.* Policy and Politics 36 (2): 261-282.

Kaeding, M. (2012). *Towards an EU Regulatory Framework for an Effective Single Market. Implementing the Many Forms of European Policy Instruments across Member States.* Wiesbaden: VS Verlag (173 pages).

Kaeding, M., Versluis E. (2014). EU Agencies as a Solution to Pan-European Implementation Problems. In: Everson, M., Monda, C, Vos, E. (eds) (2014). *European Agencies in between Institutions and Member States.* Amsterdam, Kluwer: 73-86.

Klika, C. (2015a). *Risk and the Precautionary Principle in the Implementation of REACH: The Inclusion of Substances of Very High Concern in the Candidate List.* European Journal of Risk Regulation 6 (1): 111-120.

Klika, C. (2015b). *The Implementation of the REACH Authorisation Procedure on Chemical Substances of Concern: What Kind of Legitimacy?* Politics and Governance 3 (1): 128-138.

Mastenbroek, E., Kaeding, M. (2006). *Europeanisation beyond the Goodness of Fit: Domestic Politics in the Forefront.* Comparative European Politics 4 (4): 331-354.

Mastenbroek, E., Kaeding, M. (2007). *Transcending the Goodness of Fit.* Comparative European Politics 5 (3): 342-343.

Schmälter, J. (forthcoming). *Willing and Able? A Two-Level Theory on Compliance with Civil Liberties in the EU.* Journal of European Public Policy. DOI: 10.1080/13501763.2016.1268192.

Steunenberg, B., Voermans, W., Berglund, S., Dimitrova, A., Kaeding, M., Mastenbroek, E., Meeuwse, A., Romeijn, M. (2006). *The Transposition of EC Directives: A Comparative Study of Instruments, Techniques and Processes in Six Member States.* Nijmegen: Wolf Legal Publishers.

Steunenberg, B., Kaeding, M. (2009). *'As Time Goes By': Explaining the Transposition of Maritime Directives.* European Journal of Political Research 48: 432-454.

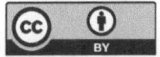

Practical Implementation in Six Member States

5

This chapter represents the core of this study and presents the main findings. The aim of this chapter is threefold. First, it offers in-depth explanations of the adverse drug reaction (ADR) reporting systems, and it describes relevant tasks and actors involved in all six countries under consideration (the United Kingdom, Finland, Poland, France, Portugal and Germany). Second, this chapter presents remaining challenges and best practices for each case as perceived by the interview partners. Third, it provides first recommendations on how to improve the existing systems in order to improve ADR reporting and help ensure public health.

5.1 ADR Reporting in the United Kingdom

5.1.1 The System

The United Kingdom has a long-established system of pharmacovigilance dating back to 1964, when the so-called Yellow Card Scheme was introduced there. Pharmacovigilance in the United Kingdom is based on a centralised system with the Medicines and Healthcare Products Regulatory Agency (MHRA) at its core.

The MHRA is the national competent authority and main regulatory body regarding medicines and pharmacovigilance and is an executive agency of the Department of Health, which is responsible for matters of legislation and finance.

Through the Yellow Card Scheme, a centralised reporting system reports on ADRs which are collected in the MHRA database. With the establishment of regional Yellow Card Centres, an element of decentralisation has been introduced. However, these centres do not play a direct role in the collection and processing of information; they aim to provide advice and training and to raise awareness (cf. below).

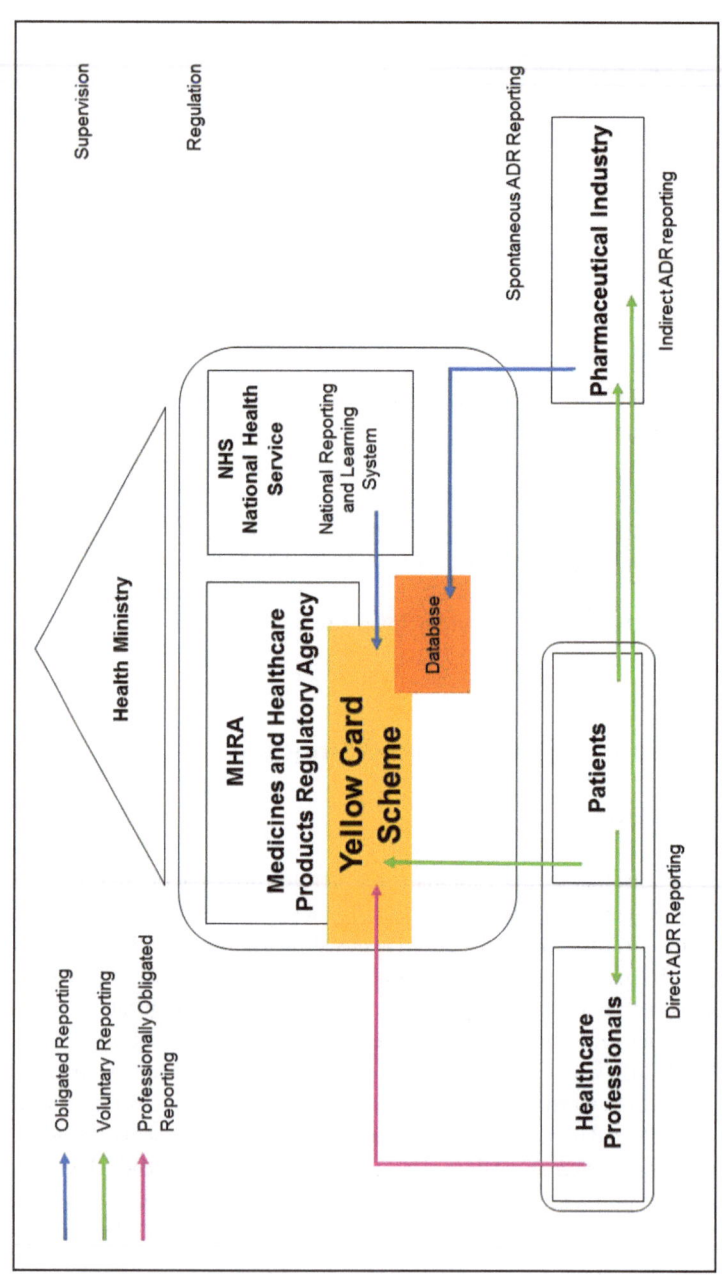

Fig. 5.1 ADR reporting in the United Kingdom (compilation by the authors)

There is no separate system for reporting ADRs arising from biologicals; the Yellow Card Scheme is used for synthetic and biological products alike. This system is shown in Fig. 5.1.

Reporting

In the 1960s, only physicians and dentists were allowed to report ADRs. However, more actors have been included over time. Since the 1990s, additional healthcare professionals (pharmacists, nurses and health visitors) have been allowed to report as well. After a pilot project, patient reporting was first introduced in 2005 and in revamped format in 2008, respectively. Hence, patient reporting in the United Kingdom was introduced before the reform of the EU pharmacovigilance system with Directive 2010/84/EU.

The way the system works is that both healthcare professionals and marketing authorisation holders submit reports to the national competent authority MHRA. Patients can report not only to the MHRA directly, but also to authorisation holders and healthcare professionals.

Healthcare professionals are not legally but professionally obligated to report ADRs and are particularly encouraged to report all serious suspected reactions to established medicines, even if the effects are already well recognised. In addition, they should report the reactions to the MHRA via the Yellow Card Scheme online form, but they can also report them to the marketing authorisation holder.

Moreover, healthcare professionals must report all suspected adverse reactions associated with black triangle products (▼), including non-serious ADRs. In the United Kingdom, all biological medicines are defined as black triangle products. Thus, even though there is no separate system for reporting ADRs related to biologicals, ADRs do receive special attention.

Marketing authorisation holders are legally obligated to report all suspected ADRs they are informed about through reports by healthcare professionals or patients or in the context of post-authorisation safety studies. Marketing authorisation holders process reports from either patients or healthcare professionals in individual case safety reports (ICSRs) and subsequently forward them to the MHRA database. Non-compliance by the industry might lead to sanctions.

Since 2005, patients are also allowed to report ADRs electronically via the Yellow Card Scheme, or by phone or regular mail to the national competent authority MHRA. In 2015, the MHRA even introduced the "Yellow Card App" for smartphones. Additionally, patients can report to healthcare professionals or the pharmaceutical industry, which must transfer the information to the MHRA database.

Furthermore, the National Health Service (NHS), as an active provider of healthcare, has its own database for medical errors and patient safety incidents, i.e. the

National Reporting and Learning System. The NHS and the national competent authority MHRA collaborate closely in order to ensure patient safety. Hence, when the National Research and Learning System identifies an ADR, the NHS forwards the information to the MHRA database.

As indicated by Fig. 5.2, healthcare professionals and marketing authorisation holders submitted roughly the same number of reports, while patient reporting remained at five to 10 percent in previous years.

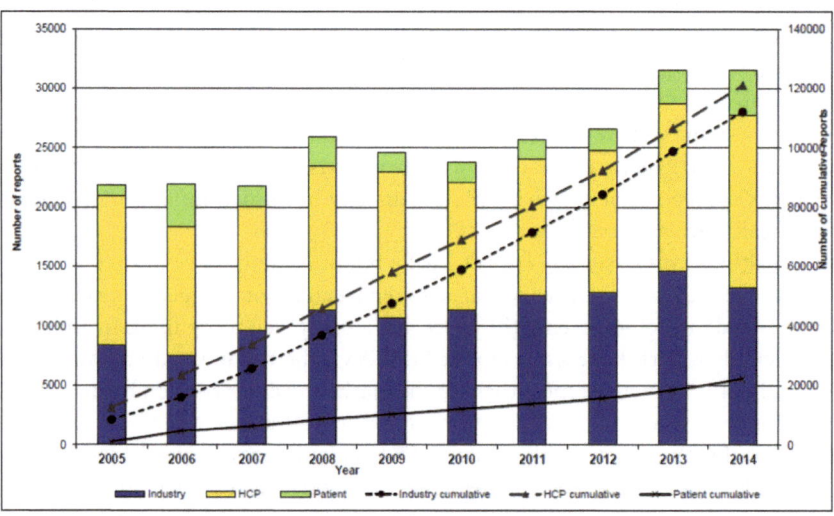

Fig. 5.2   ADR reporting by actors (2005-2014) (provided by the MHRA)

Between 2006 and 2012, there were roughly 25,000 reports per year. However, there have been substantial increases and the number of ADR reports reached 40,000 in 2015. The MHRA credits this to general promotion, integrating electronic reporting forms into clinical IT systems and the work of the Yellow Card Centres (MHRA 2016c Annual Report). In this respect, a significant increase in the reporting of both healthcare professionals and members of the public was noted by the MHRA.

Evaluation and Signal Detection

In contrast to pharmacovigilance systems in the other Member States, there is no comprehensive evaluation of reports before the stage of signal detection in the United Kingdom.

Therefore, the MHRA database consists of individual case safety reports (ICSRs) from the pharmaceutical industry, incidents from the National Report and Learning System, data from clinical trials and all ADR reports submitted via the Yellow Card Scheme. Additionally, the United Kingdom decided to include serious ICSRs from non-EU countries when ADRs relate to medicinal products authorised to be used in the United Kingdom.

As a result, the MHRA has to process extremely high numbers of ADR reports, and thus signal detection was automated. The MHRA database analyses the reports statistically with the Empirical Bayes Geometric Mean (EBGM) method, which is able to identify combinations of drug reactions that have been reported unusually frequently, and a "disproportionality score" is assigned to each combination (Foy 2015; MHRA 2016a).

The MHRA's Vigilance Intelligence and Research Group meets twice weekly. In the first meeting, all synthetic medicines with alarmingly high disproportionality scores are discussed. In the second meeting, all serious reports regarding black triangle products (▼), i.e. biologicals, are assessed, again indicating that biological medicines receive special attention in the United Kingdom.

If signals are detected in either meeting, both statistical methods and a consultation with the Commission on Human Medicines prioritise further action (MHRA 2016a). This could include deciding to update the product information leaflet, changing the dosage, issuing warnings in periodic drug safety updates or taking the product off the market.

The MHRA has 15 days to report serious cases to EMA.

5.1.2 Perceived Challenges

It is widely assumed in the literature that underreporting is inherent in spontaneous ADR reporting. In the United Kingdom, it is estimated that around 10 percent of all ADRs are reported; yet, the precise number is dependent on a variety of factors and the seriousness of the ADR (see Cousins et al. 2015).

Lack of Awareness

Evidence suggests that the general awareness about pharmacovigilance is very high among healthcare professionals and recent polls show that around 80 percent of general practitioners and pharmacists are able to identify the Yellow Card Scheme as the ADR reporting scheme (see Cousins et al. 2015). However, public awareness regarding the Yellow Card Scheme is comparably low. A survey revealed that less than 10 percent had heard of the scheme (Fortnum et al. 2012). This number seems to be fairly constant in recent years (Foy 2015) which is surprising, given that patient reporting had already been introduced in the United Kingdom in 2005. Yet, despite the long-established system of pharmacovigilance, a significant percentage of the general public seems to be unaware of it.

The interviews corroborate this evidence, pointing to a general patient unawareness regarding pharmacovigilance in general and ADR reporting in particular. Although the national competent authority MHRA is already engaged in various information campaigns (cf. below), public awareness and the knowledge of ADR reporting must be further enhanced. While the majority of people have heard of the Yellow Card Scheme through pharmacists, advertising in non-medical facilities such as public libraries has been suggested (Fortnum et al. 2012). One example of a more target-oriented approach would be to have healthcare professionals hand out information brochures when prescribing or administering drugs.

Recommendation: Awareness Raising – Patients

In order to tackle patient underreporting, European, national and regional authorities should invest in awareness-raising campaigns to increase the public knowledge about pharmacovigilance and reporting of ADRs. Authorities should raise awareness in the short term through various means of communication (e.g. websites, social media, leaflets) as well as in the long term through cooperation with schools to educate future generations.

Moreover, Member States should offer a wide range of possible communication channels, including web-based as well as paper-based formats. Both formats should be designed to be as user-friendly as possible. For web-based formats, IT solutions should be developed to guide patients through the format and to ensure the completeness of reports. All formats should be accompanied by accessible manuals written in layman's terms.

In addition to measures for facilitating patient reporting, national and regional competent authorities should also establish mechanisms to provide mandatory feedback to reporting patients.

However, unawareness is not only a challenge regarding patients, but also healthcare professionals, who often underestimate the importance of pharmacovigilance. Moreover, there seems to be a lack of sensitivity among healthcare professionals that non-serious and especially recurrent ADRs must be reported for an ongoing and expedient evaluation.

One respondent even indicated that some healthcare professionals appear to refuse engaging in ADR reporting because they consider product safety not the responsibility of practitioners but the industry producing the medications.

Recommendation: Awareness Raising – Healthcare Professionals

In order to tackle underreporting by healthcare professionals, national authorities and healthcare institutions should invest in awareness-raising campaigns to increase professional knowledge about pharmacovigilance and to sensitise relevant actors about its particular importance to ensure public health.

This lack of awareness should not come as a surprise, though, when considering academic education in this field (Smith and Webley 2013). In the United Kingdom, there is no nationwide curriculum covering pharmacovigilance in relevant studies. In undergraduate pharmacy degree programmes, pharmacovigilance is compulsory, although the amount of time dedicated to it is rather limited. And while pharmacy students discuss pharmacovigilance only sporadically, it is rather neglected for medical students. Hence, there are no mandatory classes on either pharmacovigilance or ADR reporting. It is argued that particularly causality assessment should be a basic subject in all medical schools (Edwards 2012).

Moreover, several interview partners indicated that there is not enough post-graduate training to keep up with the changing demands. They also lamented that the role of EMA and the impact of EU pharmaceuticals regulation on national pharmacovigilance is neglected (Smith and Webley 2013). We can thus assume that such neglect does not facilitate general awareness among healthcare professionals implementing EU regulation at the national level.

Awareness raising is therefore an issue in the long run in order to internalise the fact that all ADRs need to be reported for effective signal detection. Both pharmacy and medical academic programmes should include mandatory classes emphasizing the relevance of pharmacovigilance and imparting information on the practical management of ADR reporting. Additionally, the national competent authority and related research institutions should offer respective post-graduate training, constantly ensuring that practitioners understand the subject's significance and thus notify relevant actors about changing circumstances.

Recommendation: University and Post-University Training

In order to improve both the quantity and quality of ADR reports, university classes about the importance of pharmacovigilance and the need for constant ADR reporting should be mandatory for every medical and pharmacy student.

In addition, European, national or regional authorities should organise advanced post-graduate training on a regular basis to ensure that healthcare professionals acquire the necessary skills to cope with the complex task of ADR reporting.

Complexity of ADR Reporting

For biological medicines, the problems are even more severe. Even though United Kingdom law prescribes that batch numbers ought to be displayed on each package, the actual reporting of the number remains rather challenging. Healthcare professionals usually struggle with their daily routines in hospitals and do not have the time they would need to find and report the respective batch numbers. For patients, reporting the batch number is generally impossible because biologicals are generally administered directly in hospital settings, and therefore patients rarely see the respective packaging.

Recommendation: Facilitate Reporting Processes

Healthcare institutions, in line with the general health policies of their Member State, should facilitate reporting of ADRs through streamlined internal processes.

Lack of Interconnectivity

Several respondents addressed another concerning challenge, namely the use of two different electronic systems, i.e. one for managing patient data and one for reporting ADRs. This lack of connectivity between different IT systems renders the process of ADR reporting cumbersome and time-consuming and thereby severely impedes comprehensive reporting by physicians.

Note that the national competent authority MHRA already integrated the Yellow Card Scheme into two hospital systems (cf. below). This has two major advantages. First, it simplifies the reporting process because the system is able to complement large amounts of data automatically. Second, the system reminds healthcare professionals to report ADRs and makes non-reporting a more conscious decision.

Therefore, the integration of the Yellow Card Scheme into all hospital and general practitioner software programmes should be pursued further.

Recommendation: Harmonisation of IT Systems

In order to cope with information overload and to facilitate the process of submitting ADR reports, national and regional competent authorities should improve the interconnectivity of different IT systems, as for instance those of general practitioners, hospitals, pharmacies and the national competent authority's ADR reporting system.

5.1.3   Perceived Best Practices

In the United Kingdom's pharmacovigilance system, three best practices have been identified: active use of social media for awareness raising, interconnectivity regarding the Yellow Card Scheme and strong cooperation with other institutions.

Awareness Raising

The MHRA established five regional Yellow Card Centres to further promote the Yellow Card Scheme. These centres aim to raise awareness regarding ADR reporting and to improve communication between healthcare professionals and patients. In order to reach out to patients, the MHRA publishes an electronic newsletter called Drug Safety Update for interested patients.

The most important measures to date are as follows:

- In March 2013, the Yellow Card Centre of Wales launched the so-called "Yellow Card Hospital Champion Scheme" in order to increase awareness and provide further incentives for healthcare professionals to report (cf. Box 5.1).
- In 2014, a new Yellow Card website was launched as a single point of access to the reporting scheme, yielding an increase in the number of reports (MHRA 2016).
- In 2015, the 50th anniversary of the Yellow Card Scheme was celebrated with special events being held. The MHRA expects that these activities will bear fruit in the future due to systematic and cultural change regarding ADR reporting (MHRA 2016).
- In 2015, the MHRA launched the Yellow Card App (cf. Box 5.2) in order to offer a platform for information and further simplify patient reporting. Users of the smartphone app are able to create individual watch lists to receive official information and alerts about medicinal products that are relevant for them.

Furthermore, the MHRA is considerably engaged in awareness raising via social media, e.g. Facebook and Twitter. The hashtag #*ThinkPatientSafety*, for instance, is used to spread news, concerns or information via Twitter. Additionally, the MHRA not only uses social media to spread information, but also uses it as a source for signal analysis. By searching for specific keywords, statistical MHRA programmes are able to identify posts resembling ADR reports.

Although some respondents indicated a lack of sufficient pharmacovigilance training for practitioners, the MHRA is not inactive in this respect. For instance, it offers extensive guidance on pharmacovigilance and ADR reporting on its website, including free e-learning modules and particular courses for pharmacists and nurses to improve their pharmacovigilance skills. The MHRA also publishes general information about medical safety issues for all healthcare professionals as well as specific information for different specialist groups, if necessary.

Box 5.1   Best Practice: The Yellow Card App

The MHRA's Yellow Card App was introduced in 2015 as a supplement to the existing one-stop website and allows patients and healthcare professionals to directly report ADRs to the Yellow Card Scheme. The app was created in collaboration with the Innovative Medicines Initiative WEB-RADR project and is free to use for everyone who has iOS and Android. Besides ADR reporting, users can select specific medicines or vaccines to track and receive related news and alerts. More precisely, the app enables users to (1) create a watch list of medications in order to receive official news and alerts, (2) view numbers of Yellow Cards received by MHRA for medicines of interest and (3) receive immediate responses that a Yellow Card has been accepted (MHRA, iTunes store).

Interconnectivity

To begin with, most respondents are very satisfied with the MHRA's Yellow Card Scheme. It enables all actors to report ADRs and facilitates the central collection of reports, and the MHRA has already integrated the electronic Yellow Card Scheme into two out of five general practitioner software programmes. This profoundly simplifies the ADR reporting process, because physicians and pharmacists do not have to enter the relevant information twice. Additionally, this step is likely to further increase the number of ADR reports submitted by practitioners. Each time healthcare professionals intend to enter the termination of a certain medicine into the system, there will be a direct request about whether an adverse event ought to be reported. Thus, the awareness about the need to report ADRs is increased and the decision not to report becomes much more conscious.

Compared with ADR reporting in other European countries, our respondents pointed out that the United Kingdom does not have problems concerning data duplication. The MHRA has a special duplication detection programme which is able to identify reports that were submitted twice.

Box 5.2   Best Practice: Yellow Card Hospital Champion Scheme Wales

In 2011-2012, the number of Yellow Cards submitted in Wales to the MHRA (Medicines and Healthcare Products Regulatory Agency) fell by 26 percent, i.e. the lowest annual number from Wales in the past 10 years. Reports submitted by hospital pharmacists – before the leading group of reporters – fell by 37 percent as compared with the previous year. Similarly, reports from hospital physicians fell by 24 percent over the same period.

As a reaction, the Yellow Card Centre Wales (YCC Wales) submitted a proposal to the All Wales Chief Pharmacist Committee recommending the introduction of a Yellow Card Hospital Champion Scheme as an attempt to improve declining reporting rates amongst hospital-based reporters.

All health boards in Wales were asked to nominate a pharmacist or pharmacy technician as their "Yellow Card Champion". All 13 champions received training on the Yellow Card Scheme's background, ADRs and their classification, how to complete a Yellow Card, and their new role. They also attended a workshop on how to overcome barriers to completing a Yellow Card. In addition, during a 12-month period, YCC Wales sent them regular e-mails outlining the latest pharmacovigilance news. Altogether, 438 additional healthcare professionals received training on the Yellow Card Scheme at 38 sessions.

In 2013-2014, the Wales region collected 1,177 reports of suspected ADRs, an increase of 81 percent from 2012-2013. More precisely, reports from hospital pharmacists rose by 189 percent, which represents the highest number of reports ever submitted since they have been able to report via the Yellow Card Scheme. Hence, the Yellow Card Hospital Champion Scheme has been extraordinarily efficient and enabled the YCC Wales to reach a wide audience across all health boards in Wales.

Cooperation

ADR reporting in the United Kingdom is based on the collaboration of all pharma-covigilance actors, including regulatory authorities and public and private organisations, including patients' organisations. The collaborative approach is expected to facilitate awareness and learning, and it has been suggested that it could serve as a template for other countries (Cousins et al. 2015).

Moreover, the United Kingdom is among the six Member States leading the main work packages of the SCOPE implementation project, particularly leading the topics in the work packages on ADR collection, signal management, quality management systems and risk communications (MHRA 2016). Taking steps in this direction – having both healthcare professionals and patients in mind – seems vital in order to address challenges relating to the underreporting of ADRs (Edwards 2012).

The steps taken in the United Kingdom are specifically geared towards medication errors, which are included in ADR reporting since the reform of the EU pharmacovigilance system. In this respect, large healthcare providers are now required to have medical safety officers (MSOs) and medical device safety officers (MDSOs). These MSOs or MDSOs are obligated to constantly improve the medication error-reporting system in their respective organisations and to act as the main contact for NHS England and the MHRA.

These MSOs and MDSOs are automatically members of the newly founded National Medication Safety Network which was set up by MHRA and NHS England; this network is a forum for discussing potential and recognised safety issues and identifying trends and actions to enhance the safe use of medicines.

Furthermore, the MHRA organises several projects in collaboration with the NHS England in order to improve patient safety. Among others, they jointly publish "Patient Safety Alerts" to inform the public, healthcare professionals and healthcare providers about current safety issues. Recently, the MHRA has also emphasized the reporting of ADRs observed in children and young people (MHRA 2016).

The Commission on Human Medicine is an advisory non-departmental public body which works independently and is only accountable to the Department of Health. One of the Commission's sub-committees is the Expert Advisory Group for Pharmacovigilance, whose task, *inter alia*, is to issue recommendations and advice on medicinal products to the MHRA.

5.2 ADR Reporting in Finland

5.2.1 The System

The Finnish pharmacovigilance system, which was established in 1982, is headed by the Ministry of Social Affairs and Welfare. The Ministry sets the legal guidelines but is not actively involved in the system of reporting adverse drug reactions (ADRs). The key actor in the Finnish ADR reporting system is the Finnish Medicines Agency (*Lääkealan Turvallisuus – Ja Kehittämiskeskus,* or Fimea) and it collects and evaluates the ADR reports it receives from healthcare professionals, patients, the pharmaceutical industry and the National Institute for Health and Welfare (*Terveyden Ja Hyvinvoinnin Laitos,* or THL) and forwards them to the European level.

As indicated in Fig. 5.3, the Finnish ADR reporting system differentiates between synthetic medicines and vaccines; a detailed account of this framework is also described below.

Reporting

The Finnish Medicines Agency emphasizes in its guidelines that any ADR ought to be reported to the national competent authority. However, Fimea also explicitly urges reporting serious and unexpected reactions (Fimea Administrative Guideline 2/2013). Each ADR report submitted by healthcare professionals, patients or marketing authorisation holders should include the following information:

- Description of the ADR
- The suspected drug or medication involved
- Drug user data
- The course of the event
- Information about the person reporting the adverse reaction
- The product trade name and the batch number of biological products

Hence, reporting both the trade name and batch number for biologicals is explicitly required by the Finnish authorities.

Reporting by healthcare professionals. In Finland, "persons authorised to prescribe or supply drugs *are advised* to report to Fimea any adverse reaction they find or suspect in association with the use of drugs" (Fimea Guideline 2/2010, emphasis added). Thus, healthcare professionals are not legally required to report ADRs related to synthetic products, although they are legally obligated to report ADRs resulting from vaccines.

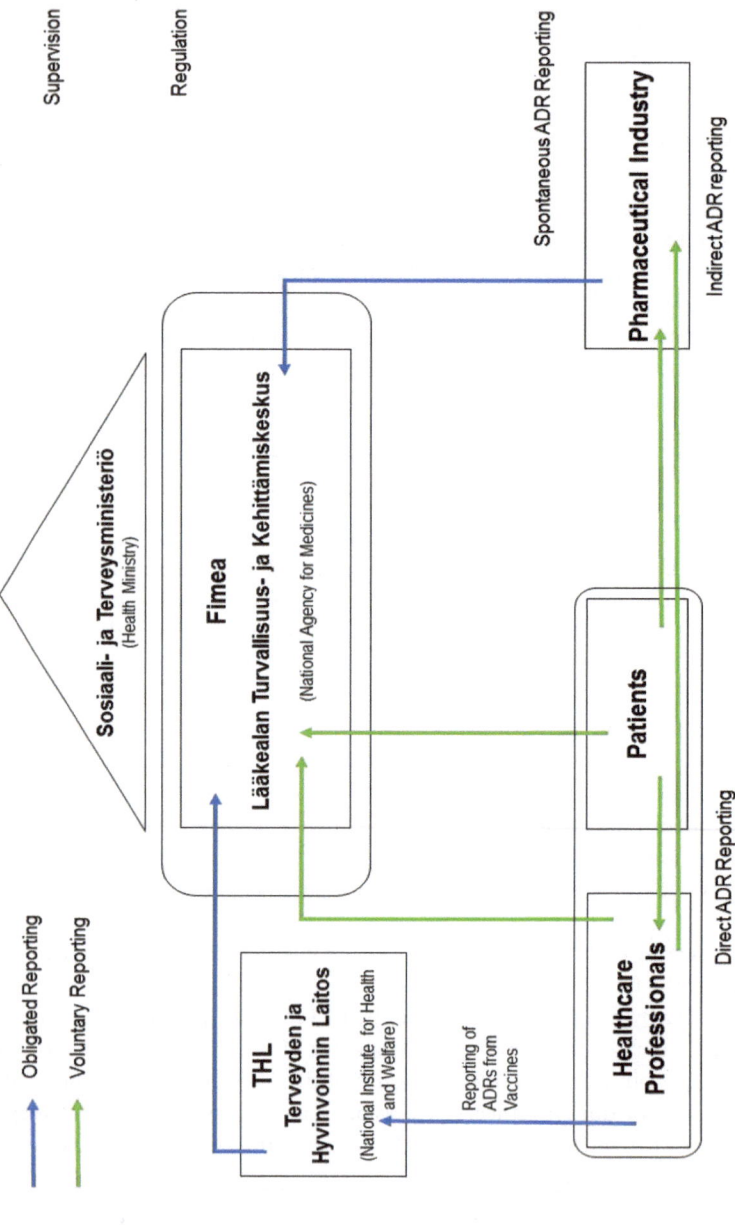

Fig. 5.3 ADR reporting in Finland (compilation by the authors)

ADRs of synthetic products should be reported to Fimea. Physicians and pharmacists can report via regular mail or download an online form on Fimea's homepage and then submit the completed form there. In order to report electronically, however, healthcare professionals need access to FIMnet; physicians and pharmacists receive their FIMnet user ID through membership in their respective professional associations.

Since 2012, nurses are also allowed to report. Yet, unlike physicians and pharmacists, they do not have access to FIMnet. Instead, they must print out an online form and then submit it via regular mail.

As already described above, ADRs caused by vaccines are treated differently. According to the Finnish Communicable Diseases Act (583/1986, 12b), "Healthcare professionals *must* notify all identified or suspected adverse effects of a vaccine that have come to their knowledge" (emphasis added). Here, instead of being advised to contact Fimea, healthcare professionals are required to inform the National Institute for Health and Welfare and the institute subsequently sends the respective data to Fimea.

Besides reporting to the national competent authority, all healthcare professionals, i.e. physicians, pharmacists and nurses, are allowed to inform the respective marketing authorisation holder about ADRs. The marketing authorisation holders are then legally obligated to forward the reports to Fimea. In the case of non-compliance, marketing authorisation holders risk the launch of infringement procedures or the imposition of sanctions. Thus, while healthcare professionals are only legally obligated to report ADRs related to vaccines, the pharmaceutical industry is under the obligation to report all adverse events to Fimea.

Patient reporting. Since the transposition of Directive 2010/84/EU in 2012, patients are also allowed to report ADRs. Similar to nurses, they cannot report electronically but need to contact Fimea via regular mail. In addition, patients can consult with their treating physician, pharmacist or the respective marketing authorisation holder in order to notify them about suspected ADRs. In fact, in their "Guidelines on Adverse Drug Reporting", Fimea specifies that it prefers that patients get in touch with healthcare professionals before sending reports directly to the national competent authority, arguing that reporting cannot be considered a substitute for consulting an expert (Fimea Guideline 2/2010).

Fig. 5.4 indicates that in 2015 Fimea received most reports by physicians, i.e. 1,230. Physicians especially report reactions to new medicines and those that are under special surveillance (e.g. black triangle products (▼)). In comparison, nurses filed 700 reports, which is an impressive number when taking into account that they must always jump through the bureaucratic hoops of printing the forms and sending them by regular mail. Pharmacists and patients submitted 270 and 400 reports, respectively. Thus, in 2015 a total number of 2,600 reports were submitted to Fimea (excluding reports by marketing authorisation holders).

Evaluation and Signal Detection

All reports received by Fimea are entered into the national Adverse Reaction Register. The data is coded by specialists and then medically evaluated by healthcare professionals and a database. Finally, after evaluation, Fimea forwards the details of all ADR reports via regular mail to the respective marketing authorisation holders, EMA and the WHO.

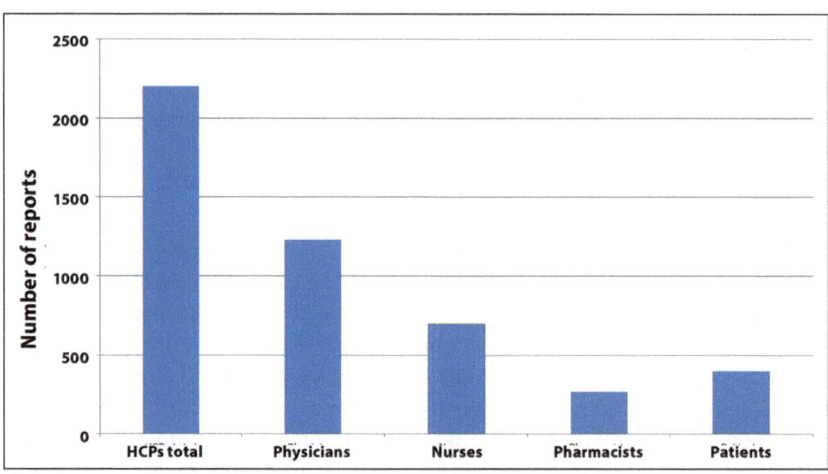

Fig. 5.4   ADR reporting by actors in 2015 (provided by Fimea)

5.2.2 Perceived Challenges

Several challenges have been identified by our interviewees, especially regarding Fimea's decision-making power, the actors who are able to report and the connection between different healthcare IT systems.

First, some respondents mentioned that they consider Fimea's dominance in the Finnish pharmacovigilance system problematic. Even though the agency is officially operating under the Ministry of Social Affairs and Welfare, it is *de facto* independent.

Thus, the result is that only very few people are responsible for making all decisions regarding pharmacovigilance and ADR reporting without elaborate supervision.

Lack of Awareness

Generally, our respondents were rather satisfied with the quantity of reports submitted to Fimea. Some of them, however, indicated that healthcare professionals are too focused on reporting serious and new ADRs. Recurrent and non-serious ADRs, they claim, are largely neglected and usually unrecorded.

Recommendation: Awareness Raising – Healthcare Professionals

In order to tackle underreporting by healthcare providers, national authorities and healthcare institutions should invest in awareness-raising campaigns to increase professional knowledge about pharmacovigilance and sensitise relevant actors about its importance to ensure public health.

Additionally, and considering Fimea's particular emphasis on the reporting of serious ADRs, reducing this emphasis from the guidelines on ADR reporting should be considered. Instead, more prominence should be given to reporting all ADRs, including recurrent and non-serious reactions.

Furthermore, our respondents were divided on the particular importance Fimea assigns to physicians and pharmacists, namely the only actors in the Finnish ADR system who are able to report electronically. Both patients and nurses have to resort to regular mail in order to report ADRs. This was perceived as rather unconstructive by several interviewees because nurses are particularly well trained regarding medication and identifying potential ADRs. Thus, *prima facie* there is no reasonable explanation why nurses are excluded from reporting electronically. Additionally, physicians are usually rather overworked which might render them unwilling to engage in ADR reporting. An additional group of reporters would presumably facilitate the process for all actors engaged.

Supposedly, this issue can be traced back to a more cultural explanation, i.e. a top-down relationship between physicians and nurses which has been customary in Finland for generations. In the Finnish healthcare system, physicians are still perceived as the most relevant actors and this status considerably impedes cooperation with other healthcare professionals. Thus, facilitating ADR reporting for nurses without medical confirmation from physicians would contradict the Finnish top-down relationship and impair the perceived "dominant" status of physicians.

Recommendation: Facilitate Reporting by Nurses

The prestige and perceived infallibility of physicians hinders the development of the Finnish pharmacovigilance system. Thus, cultural changes are necessary to adjust the level of competence and strengthen the appreciation of nurses to improve the process of reporting. The working relationship should be considered as cooperative rather than competitive. Nurses should therefore be enabled to report electronically, as they are sufficiently educated and would significantly reduce the duties and workload of physicians.

Yet not only nurses are impeded from reporting, but also patients are impeded; they have to go through the bureaucratic hurdles of searching, printing and mailing a reporting form to Fimea instead of using an electronic form. Accordingly, Finnish patients need to be very determined if they want to report an ADR to the national competent authority.

Despite this, most of our Finnish interview partners strongly support this method. They contend that reports submitted by physicians and pharmacists are of better quality regarding both completeness and content, while the majority of consumer reports include non-serious or already-listed events which these partners consider irrelevant from a signal detection point of view. Hence, impeding patient reports has been a conscious decision and is not perceived as a challenge by the relevant actors in Finland.

However, what is considered problematic is that patients are not informed about the possibility to report at all. Even if Fimea prefers not to be directly contacted by patients, the public ought to be informed about the possibility to report via consulting physicians and pharmacists.

Recommendation: Awareness Raising – Patients

In order to tackle underreporting by patients, Fimea, the national competent authority, should invest in awareness-raising campaigns to increase the public knowledge about pharmacovigilance and reporting of adverse drug reactions.

Authorities should raise awareness in the short term through various means of communication (e.g. websites, social media, leaflets) as well as in the long term through cooperation with schools to educate future generations.

Moreover, Member States should offer a wide range of possible communication channels, including web-based and paper-based formats. Both types of formats

---

should be designed to be as user-friendly as possible. For web-based formats, IT solutions should be developed to guide patients through the format and to ensure the completeness of reports. All formats should be accompanied by accessible manuals written in layman's terms.

Lack of Interconnectivity

ADR reporting for healthcare professionals has been identified as very time-consuming, particularly because there is no IT connection between Fimea's ADR reporting system and the various systems recording patient data. Therefore, our respondents regard more IT connectivity between different healthcare systems as a necessary step to facilitate ADR reporting. Thus, although most healthcare professionals are aware of the importance of reporting, they are impeded from doing so by the rather cumbersome reporting system.

However, it should be noted that connecting reporting systems with systems storing patient data is currently rather challenging in Finland. The responsibility to organise healthcare services is in the hands of 300 municipalities. Because each municipality individually decides which patient record system to use, there are numerous systems for recording patient data which considerably exacerbates their connection and the connection to Fimea's ADR reporting system.

In the years to come, the Finnish authorities plan to implement a significant healthcare reform aiming to transfer responsibilities from the municipal level to the regional level. Our respondents expect that afterwards the quality of patient record systems is likely to increase and render the connection to ADR reporting systems easier.

Recommendation: Harmonisation of IT Systems

In order to cope with information overload and to facilitate the process of submitting ADR reports, national and regional competent authorities should improve interconnectivity of IT systems, including those of general practitioners, hospitals, pharmacies and the national competent authority's ADR reporting system.

5.2.3 Perceived Best Practices

Awareness Raising

The importance of reporting ADRs is mainly accepted by physicians and pharmacists in Finland, even though it is not always easy for them to integrate ADR reporting into their daily working routine.

This can be mainly attributed to a very elaborate education system for healthcare professionals regarding pharmacovigilance. Pharmacovigilance and ADR reporting are part of the mandatory curriculum of both physicians and pharmacists. Moreover, pharmacists who are in contact with patients are required to have more advanced university degrees. Less-educated people are not allowed to work at the counter or to have direct contact with patients and are thus not allowed to report.

Additionally, Fimea offers voluntary advanced training for physicians, nurses and medical students, for example at the HUS hospital in Helsinki. During those training sessions, current trends, ADR reports and signals are thoroughly discussed, leading to high-quality reports.

Reporting of Batch Numbers

ADR reports related to vaccines need to contain not only the brand name, but also the product's batch number. Interestingly, there are barely any problems concerning missing information. As Table 5.1 reveals, most vaccines that have been in the register in 2015 have been identified by their batch number.

Tab. 5.1   How vaccines are identified (provided by THL) (in percent)

	2012	2013	2014	2015
Vaccines identified	98.7	99.1	99.4	99.7
...by batch number	93.9	95.4	96.3	97.2
...by trade name	3.8	3.0	2.9	2.2
Vaccines *not* identified	1.3	0.9	0.5	0.3

Interconnectivity

Finally, another positive example is the electronic connection between the IT systems of physicians and pharmacists. This IT connectivity allows physicians to ensure that patients pick up the prescribed drugs at the pharmacies. Even though this connectivity could be further improved, it is a promising starting point that should be considered by other pharmacovigilance systems across the EU.

5.3 ADR Reporting in Poland

5.3.1 The System

The Polish health ministry, although responsible for the health system's financing and its resources, only fulfils a supervisory role in the ADR reporting scheme and is not involved in its daily routines.

The Office for Registration of Medicinal Products, Medical Devices and Biocidal Products (Urząd Rejestracji Produktów Leczniczych, Wyrobów Medycznych i Produktów Biobójczych, or URPL) is the Polish national competent authority for the reception and evaluation of all submitted ADR reports. Moreover, the URPL is also responsible for forwarding the relevant reports to European and international databases. It is affiliated with the national health ministry but acts largely independently from it. The URPL is also responsible for educating and training healthcare professionals as well as supervising the pharmaceutical industry. In addition, the URPL informs health professionals about new developments in pharmacovigilance and issues warnings. Because it is technically and professionally competent, it is able to influence political discussions on pharmacovigilance and initiates reforms in close cooperation with the health ministry.

Fig. 5.5 illustrates ADR reporting in Poland.

Reporting

Reporting by healthcare professionals. Healthcare professionals, including not only physicians, pharmacists and nurses, but also dentists, nurses, midwives, laboratory diagnosticians, paramedics and pharmaceutical technicians, are legally obligated to report any ADRs; however, there are no anticipated penalties for not doing so. Healthcare professionals must complete reports and submit them either to the national competent authority URPL or to the marketing authorisation holders in question. Moreover, they need to act as contact people for further questions and must provide additional information if required. Reports can be submitted by e-mail, fax, through regular mail or online.

Reporting by marketing authorisation holders. The pharmaceutical industry, which includes the marketing authorisation holders as well as the medicinal product manufacturers, is also legally obligated to submit reports on ADRs to the URPL. However, in contrast to healthcare professionals, actors in the pharmaceutical industry face non-reporting penalties ranging from paying severe fines to imprisonment.

Patient reporting. The patients, in contrast to the two former actors in the system, can submit their reports voluntarily and have three reporting options. They can either inform a healthcare professional (mostly the responsible doctor or pharmacist)

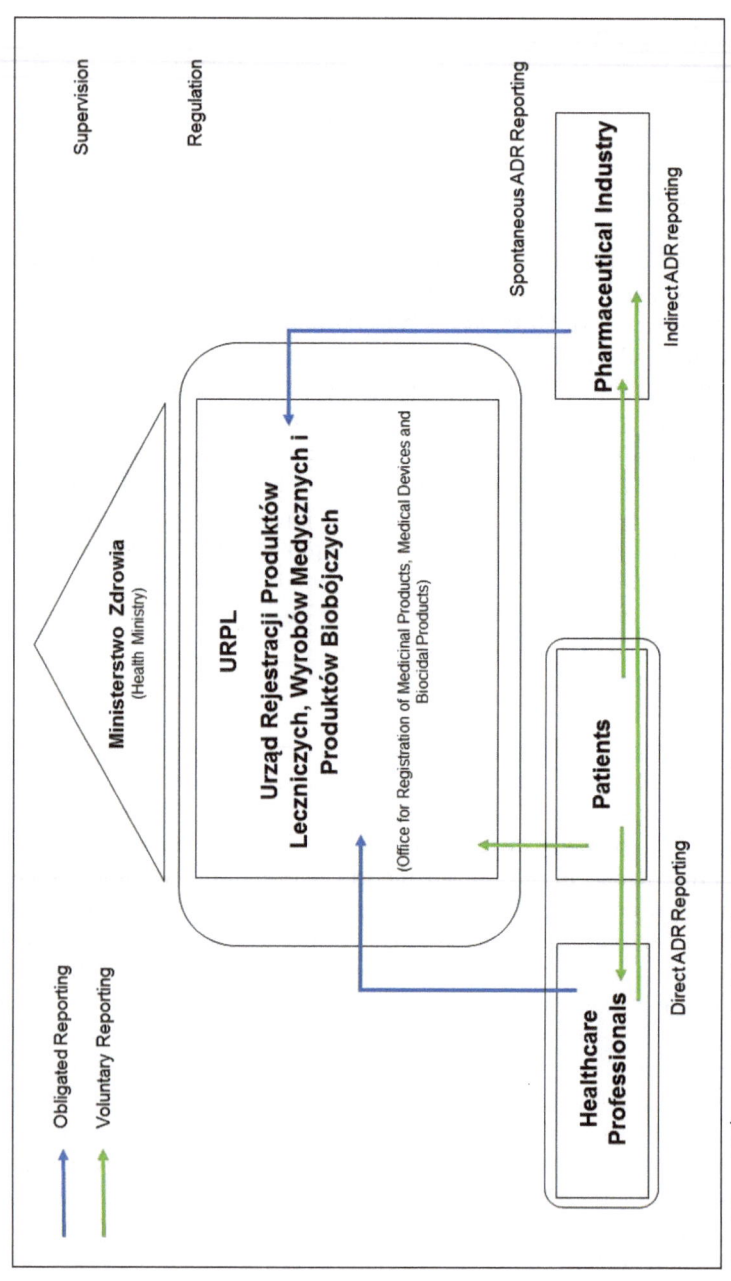

Fig. 5.5   ADR reporting in Poland (compilation by the authors)

or the marketing authorisation holder in question. Moreover, the patient also has the option to report the ADR directly to the URPL office. The report can be submitted by e-mail, fax, through regular mail or online.

Evaluation and Signal Detection

The national competent authority URPL receives the ADR reports from patients, healthcare professionals and the pharmaceutical industry alike and carries out the causality assessment of the reported incidents, evaluating them scientifically in order to detect signals. The agency is also able to contact the reporters for additional questions or to fill in missing information. Once the report is completed and scientifically evaluated, it is forwarded to EudraVigilance and the database of the WHO. Moreover, the agency sends feedback to the reporters.

The ADR reporting scheme in general does not differentiate between biological and non-biological medicines. However, there is one exception to this rule: Vaccines and possible negative side effects stemming from vaccinations are treated in a separate system. In Poland, vaccines are administered by healthcare professionals mostly working in centres responsible for public health issues. Therefore, the majority of the vaccines are given by personnel who deal with vaccines on a daily basis and are both well-informed about possible negative side effects and well-trained to identify possible symptoms. If any ADR is detected, a report is submitted to the responsible Regional Sanitary Board, which is obligated to send a copy of the report to the URPL. In the case of serious ADRs, the Regional Sanitary Board has to inform the State Sanitary Inspectorate which in turn forwards the report to the Chief Sanitary Inspectorate (c.f. Fig. 5.6).

5.3.2 Perceived Challenges

One of the challenges of the Polish pharmacovigilance system is underreporting, although the overall reporting quality is perceived as being good. A number of reasons for the non-reporting of ADRs have been identified and are discussed in the following paragraphs.

Lack of Awareness

Lack of time and awareness, and the fact that the reporting procedure is perceived as being complex and burdensome, lead to non-reporting among healthcare professionals. Moreover, a strong hierarchical order within hospitals, which is part of the Polish social culture, further impedes efficient reporting. There is the widespread misconception that ADRs only occur in the case of medication errors, and thus healthcare professionals are afraid of damaging their own reputations by reporting ADRs. Medical supervisors and management boards are also considered to be rather restrictive about reporting adverse reactions, trying to avoid reports because others' possible misbehaviour medical errors could be exposed, possibly leading to legal consequences such as claims for damages.

Recommendation: Awareness Raising – Healthcare Professionals

In order to tackle underreporting by healthcare providers, national authorities and healthcare institutions should invest in awareness-raising campaigns to increase professional knowledge about pharmacovigilance and sensitise relevant actors about its particular importance to ensure public health.

Additionally, training should include practical and legal counselling in order to alleviate the fear of litigation. While respecting national diversity in health-related and legal terms, it is important to recognise that fault-based systems are a significant impediment to ADR reporting. A general and cautious recommendation would be to enable healthcare professionals to report ADRs without fear of liability. This could be pursued not only by practical and legal counselling for healthcare professionals, but also by legal means through strengthening confidentiality or setting up compensation schemes for patients' claims.

The Polish pharmacovigilance system faces the insufficient education of professionals on the topic, because pharmacovigilance is not taught in a coordinated manner at the medical and pharmaceutical faculties at the country's universities. Instead, education and training for students remain dependent on the personal engagement of single professors. A systematic organisation for training is also lacking for healthcare professionals. In addition, the options for continuous training and professional development programmes are very limited.

Recommendation: University and Post-University Training

In order to improve both the quantity and quality of ADR reports, university classes about the importance of pharmacovigilance and the need for constant ADR reporting should be mandatory for every medical and pharmacy student.

In addition, the URPL should organise advanced post-graduate training on a regular basis to ensure that healthcare professionals acquire the necessary skills to cope with the complex task of ADR reporting.

The lack of a sound academic and professional network of pharmacovigilance in Poland is also perceived as a challenge to the system. Although a number of institutes and organisations are engaged in the national pharmacovigilance system and research in this field, there is only a very limited, informal exchange of information and study results. Experience and new insights can get lost because of the lack of academic and professional interconnections.

Patients are not sufficiently educated on pharmacovigilance and know very little about the possibilities to report ADRs. Although first steps have been taken to educate the public about pharmacovigilance and adverse events (cf. Box 5.3), many gaps remain. Moreover, better-educated patients can also possibly monitor healthcare professionals and motivate them towards more active ADR reporting. The patients' advantage is that the repercussions of the hierarchical hospital system and possible professional consequences do not affect them.

Recommendation: Awareness Raising – Patients

In order to tackle underreporting by patients, the URPL should invest in awareness-raising campaigns to increase the public knowledge about pharmacovigilance and the reporting of ADRs.

Authorities should raise awareness in the short term through various means of communication (e.g. websites, social media, leaflets) as well as in the long term through cooperation with schools to educate future generations.

Moreover, Member States should offer a wide range of possible communication channels, including web-based and paper-based formats. Both web-based and paper-based formats should be designed to be as user-friendly as possible. For web-based formats, IT solutions should be developed to guide patients through the format and to ensure the completeness of reports. All formats should be accompanied by accessible manuals written in layman's terms.

Incomplete Reports

The Polish pharmacovigilance scheme is relatively inexperienced in tracking and using biologicals. Because the Polish pharmaceutical industry is focused on producing generic drugs, professionals and also predominantly the national competent authorities are rather inexperienced in monitoring and supervising biological medicines. Hence, the ADR reporting scheme does not differentiate between biological and non-biological medicines, except for vaccinations. Thus, not only risks, but also benefits of biological medicines can be underestimated and warning signs can be overlooked due to inexperience in the field. Moreover, these both lead to problems in ADR reporting. Due to the relative inexperience with biologicals and a lack of training, batch numbers are not coherently reported and traceability is hampered.

Recommendation: Training on Biological Products

European, national or regional authorities should organise advanced post-graduate training on a regular basis to ensure that healthcare professionals acquire the necessary skills to cope with the complex task of ADR reporting.

In order to tackle underreporting of batch numbers and thereby facilitate the correct and timely traceability of biologicals, healthcare professionals should receive additional training to both increase awareness about the particular relevance of ADR reporting related to biologicals and to acquire the necessary skills to do so.

Budgetary Constraints

The national competent authority URPL has very limited personnel capacities and limited financial resources which both restrain its scope of actions; each year, the number of submitted reports increases while the workforce remains the same. Hence, reports cannot be evaluated as fast as would be desired. In addition, ADR reporting by telephone cannot be done because it would take too much time.

Recommendation: Sufficient Financial Means for Relevant Actors

National and regional competent authorities working under the auspices of national ministries should be endowed with sufficient financial means to fulfil their functions. Likewise, healthcare institutions should be endowed with sufficient means. Sound finances enable healthcare institutions to rely on a stronger workforce which reduces the workload of individual healthcare professionals and increases the possibility of extended the reporting of ADRs.

5.3.3 Perceived Best Practices

Awareness Raising

The URPL aims at spreading information and raising awareness in the general public, not only to educate patients, but also to reach healthcare professionals. The agency uses different social media accounts (cf. Box 5.3), and has produced two animated movies (URPL 2016) which explain how to report ADRs and offer training for professionals.

Box 5.3   Best Practice: URPL on social media

The Polish URPL is very active on social media with a Twitter and Facebook account as well as a YouTube channel. The authority posts news, interesting insights and information on pharmacovigilance, among other URPL topics. It uses the hashtag *#safedrug* to promote knowledge about ADR reporting and pharmacovigilance. Moreover, URPL published two animated movies which explain how to report an ADR and adverse events to the authority (URPL 2014, 2015).

Reporting System for Vaccines

A positive example, especially for the ADR reporting of biological medicines, is the reporting scheme for negative effects deriving from vaccines (cf. Fig. 5.6). The system is different from the general ADR reporting scheme because it follows a decentralised approach for reporting vaccine ADRs. Physicians and feldshers are legally obligated to report ADRs stemming from vaccines to the Regional Sanitary Board. Other healthcare professionals can voluntarily file an ADR report but are not obligated to do so.

The Regional Sanitary Board receives the ADR report, adds it to a database that stores ADR reports on vaccines for 10 years, and is obligated to forward a copy of the report to the national competent authority URPL. With a serious ADR event, the regional unit has to inform the State Sanitary Board (*Wojewodzki Inspektorat Sanitarny*, or WIS) within an hour after receiving the report. The WIS in turn informs the Chief Sanitary Inspectorate (*Główny Inspektorat Sanitarny*, or GIS). The GIS keeps records of all ADRs caused by vaccines and publishes a yearly report. This system enables a close monitoring of ADRs resulting from vaccinations, and it ensures high numbers of reporting because it is well-known and broadly accepted among professionals. In addition, batch number reporting functions well because the personnel is trained accordingly.

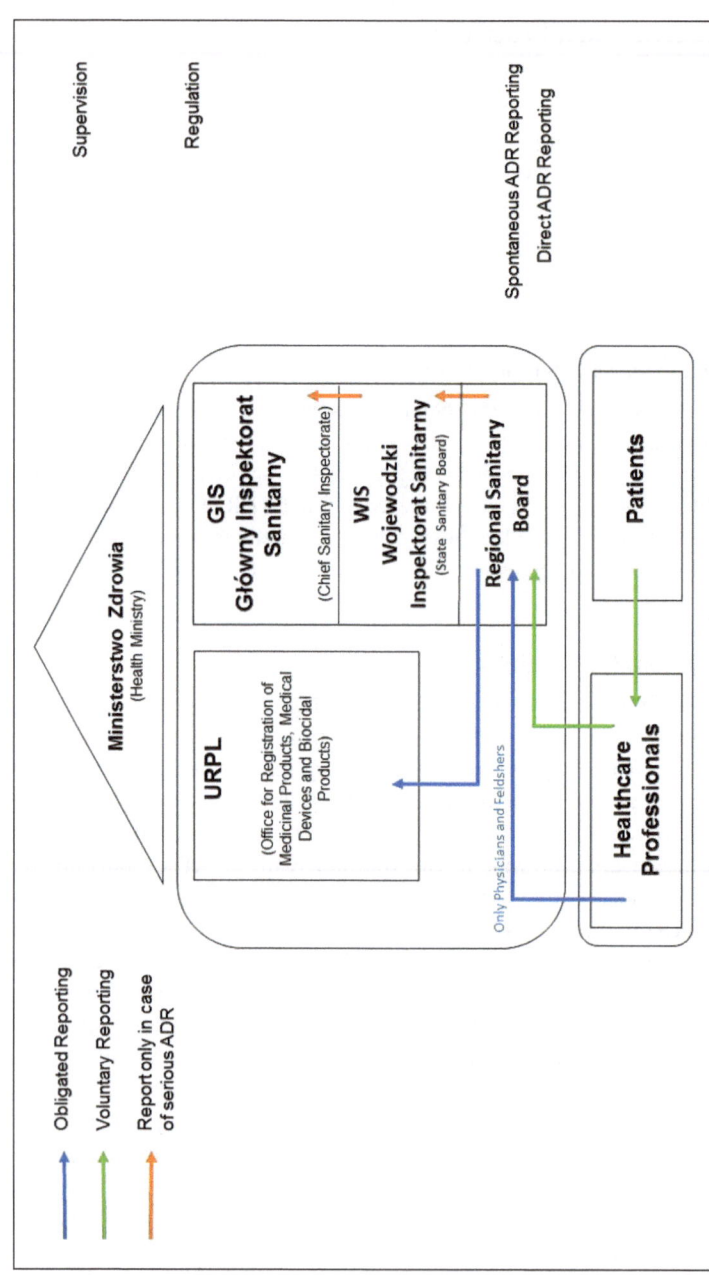

Fig. 5.6   Reporting of ADRs stemming from vaccines (compilation by the authors)

5.4 ADR Reporting in France

5.4.1 The System

Since 1973, pharmacovigilance in France has been organised by a decentralised network of 31 regional centres (*Centres Régionaux de Pharmacovigilance*, or CRPVs) and the national competent authority, namely the Agency for Drug Safety and Health Products (*Agence Nationale de Sécurité de Médicament et des Produits de Santé*, or ANSM). While the CRPVs are in charge of data collection and validation, the ANSM is responsible for data evaluation and overall decision-making processes. The French Ministry for Health and Social Security is responsible for the legal framework, finances, and the overall supervision of the French pharmacovigilance system.

The process of adverse drug reaction (ADR) reporting in France is illustrated by Fig. 5.7 and explained in the following sections. Currently, there is no separate system for reporting ADRs arising from biologicals, so the system outline below refers to the reporting of both synthetic and biological medicines.

Reporting

Reporting by healthcare professionals. Healthcare professionals constitute one of the major pillars of the French ADR reporting system. Physicians, dentists, pharmacists and midwives are legally obligated to report any ADR they encounter (*Loi de l'etat 2011-2012 du 29 décembre 2011 relative au renforcement de la sécurité sanitaire du médicament et des produits de santé*); non-compliance can lead to three years of imprisonment and a fine of up to €45,000 (ibid., Article 28).

According to French legislation, healthcare professionals must file a report to the regional CRPV where the patient is based that contains all the necessary information. Reports can be submitted via regular mail, e-mail, via an online form or by fax. During the evaluation procedure in the regional centres, healthcare professionals act as contact points and must be open to follow-up questions from the regional CRPV's experts.

Reporting by the pharmaceutical industry. In addition, the pharmaceutical industry has the legal obligation to file a report on every ADR it is informed about and any failure to comply can result in a fine of up to €150,000 and two years' imprisonment (*Code de la santé publique*, Article L. 5421-5). The respective marketing authorisation holders must send the report directly to the national competent authority ANSM, again by regular mail, e-mail or via an online form.

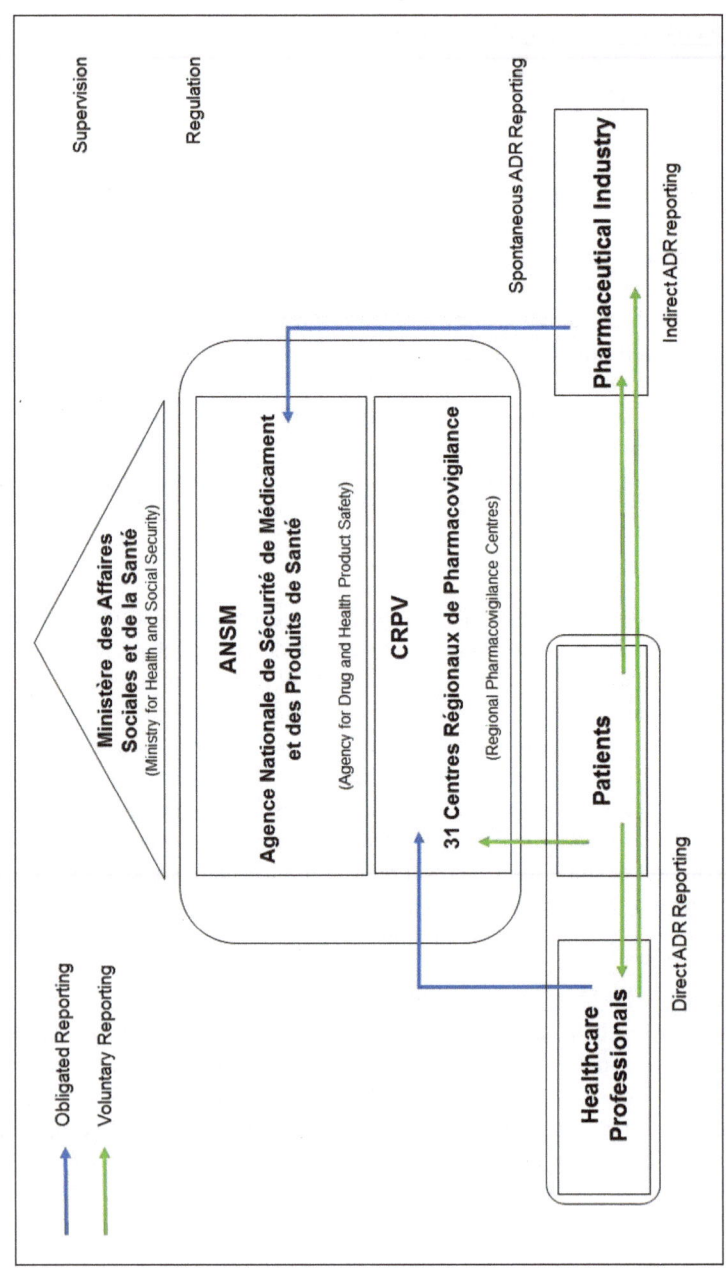

Fig. 5.7 ADR reporting in France (compilation by the authors)

Patient reporting. Finally, since June 2011, patients have also been empowered to report ADRs, although they can report on a voluntary basis. If a patient suspects an ADR, he or she has different options for reporting. First, the patient can choose to inform the regional pharmacovigilance centres or the ANSM by mail, fax and often via an online form. Interestingly, a study by Health Action International (Santos n.d.: 13) found that "in France, about half of the regional pharmacovigilance centres did not appear to have their own website to report ADRs" and only very few were found to allow direct online reporting. Further, a patient has the possibility to directly contact the marketing authorisation holder for the medicinal product in question. Third, the patient can consult a healthcare professional for advice and assistance in reporting.

Some regular centres provide feedback to reporters. As Health Action International (Santos n.d.: 8) summarised: "Toulouse, for example, sends a letter to patients who report an ADR. It includes a summary of the report and its assessment and the extent to which the report has been transferred to the national database. Relevant scientific publications can also be attached".

Evaluation and Signal Detection

All reports submitted by healthcare professionals and patients are collected by the 31 regional pharmacovigilance centres which are located in university hospitals all over the country. The regional CRPVs' pharmacovigilance units scientifically evaluate the reports and conduct the causality assessments. After verification by CRPV experts, the reports are collected in the French pharmacovigilance database (FPD) which is hosted by the ANSM; the reports submitted by marketing authorisation holders are directly sent to the FPD.

There are monthly meetings between the heads of the regional centres and the ANSM's Technical Committee (Caron et al. 2014). This committee is responsible for collecting and evaluating further information about ADRs, assessing the evaluated reports for trends in order to detect larger signals and, subsequently, forwarding these to the ANSM's general director. If deemed necessary, the committee forwards their findings to the EMA and the international database of the WHO.

In 2014, the ANSM received 46,497 ADR reports (initial and follow-up) from the regional centres, 1,983 of which were submitted by patients (ANSM Annual Report 2015).

5.4.2   Perceived Challenges

The French pharmacovigilance system is suffering from the aftermath of the so-called Mediator scandal which cost more than 2,000 deaths as a consequence of serious delays in ADR reporting and an inadequate reaction from the national competent authority (cf. Box 5.4). Many of our respondents emphasised that this scandal has still not been entirely processed by the French pharmacovigilance system and the actors involved. Instead, the respondents pointed out that many systematic difficulties remain, considerably impeding efficient and independent pharmacovigilance. For instance, it is not explicitly prohibited to work for the pharmaceutical industry and to be a member of the national competent authority at the same time. Consequently, conflicts of interest of ANSM committee members regarding the monitoring medicinal products are still present. And even though conflicts of interests formally need to be declared, there is no penalty for not doing so.

All of our respondents indicated that the French pharmacovigilance system currently faces numerous challenges. Again, underreporting is considered one of the major weaknesses. Several reasons for this have been identified by our interviewees and are discussed in the following sections.

Lack of Awareness

First, the relevant actors in the French pharmacovigilance system are often unaware either of their obligation to report ADRs or the importance of reporting ADRs, especially those arising from biological medicines. This leads many healthcare professionals to completely neglect this issue in the course of their daily routines.

Recommendation: Awareness Raising – Healthcare Professionals

In order to tackle underreporting by healthcare providers, national authorities and healthcare institutions should invest in awareness-raising campaigns to increase professional knowledge about pharmacovigilance and sensitise relevant actors about its importance to ensure public health.

This training should especially increase understanding about the particular relevance of ADR reporting related to biologicals and impart the necessary skills to do so.

Complexity and Lack of Interconnectivity

In addition, several interview partners mentioned that the workload of healthcare professionals was already considerable; therefore, healthcare professionals often refuse to engage in ADR reporting, perceiving it as a time-consuming and complex task which is difficult to integrate into daily routines. Administrative hurdles also make it difficult for healthcare professionals to report. First, reports need to be submitted via a separate online portal, and thus information needs to be collected from different IT systems. Patients must also be informed. In addition, practitioners are expected to be available for any follow-up questions from the regional centres. In summary, ADR reporting turns into a long process which cannot simply be reduced to the mere submission of a report.

Recommendation: Facilitate ADR Reporting Processes

Healthcare institutions, in line with the French general health policies, should facilitate ADR reporting through streamlined internal processes.

In order to cope with information overload and to facilitate the process of submitting ADR reports, national and regional competent authorities should improve the interconnectivity of IT systems, such as those of general practitioners, hospitals, pharmacies and the ANSM's ADR reporting system.

Additionally, all stakeholders at the national level should improve mechanisms of cooperation. This not only includes competent authorities, but also industry and patients' associations as well as research and training facilities such as universities.

Box 5.4   **The 2009 Mediator scandal in France**

From 1976 to 2009, the French manufacturer *Laboratoires Servier* sold the drug benfluorex under the brand name Mediator on the French market. The product was originally designed to control the weight of patients suffering from diabetes or obesity. However, it was often prescribed off-label to people with no other medical indications as an appetite suppressant for facilitating weight loss. In the early 2000s, the first studies found that the medication causes cardiac valve damage and pulmonary hypertension. Despite repeated warning signs and studies pointing at the causality between taking the drug and cardiac illnesses, however, neither the French authorities nor *Laboratoires Servier* reacted. Only in 2009 did the national agency AFSSAPS (now the national competent authority ANSM) finally ban the drug and investigations were started by an independent commission. The final report argues that both the company as well as the country's regulatory system are responsible for this medical scandal, which caused an estimated 2,000 deaths and led to many more patients being hospitalised with cardiac problems (Mullard 2011; Casassus 2016).

Fear of Litigation

ADRs can occur despite medications being correctly prescribed and correctly administered. However, our respondents indicated that French healthcare professionals still often consciously avoid reporting ADRs due to a fear of litigation and loss of reputation. Reporting an ADR is still often considered akin to confessing to a medical error.

Recommendation: Legal Counselling

The previously suggested pharmacovigilance training should include both practical and legal counselling in order to alleviate the fear of litigation. While respecting national diversity in health-related and legal terms, it is important to recognise that fault-based systems are an important impediment to the reporting of ADRs. A general and cautious recommendation is to enable healthcare professionals to report ADRs without fear of liability. This could be pursued not only by practical and legal counselling for healthcare professionals, but also by legal means through strengthening confidentiality or setting up compensation schemes for patients' claims.

Incomplete Reports

Another closely related problem identified by our interviewees is the weak quality of submitted reports. Frequently, brand names or relevant patient information is either inaccurate or completely omitted, and reported batch numbers appear to be the exception, especially with biological medicines. The varying quality of ADR reports thus exacerbates sound causality assessments and often renders them impossible. This emphasizes the need for a separate system regarding the reporting of biological medicines in order to guarantee sound monitoring and an appropriate risk-benefit assessment.

Recommendation: Training on Biological Products

European, national or regional authorities should organise advanced post-graduate training on a regular basis to ensure that healthcare professionals acquire the necessary skills to cope with the complex task of reporting ADRs.

In order to tackle underreporting of batch numbers and thereby facilitate the correct and timely traceability of biologicals, healthcare professionals should receive additional training to both increase awareness about the particular relevance of ADR reporting related to biologicals and to acquire the necessary skills to do so.

Budgetary Constraints

Finally, public health seems not to be an economic priority. This is visible not only from the Mediator scandal, but also in the dependencies faced by the regional centres that rely on financing from the state budget and political priorities set by the Health Ministry. Thus, regional budgets are rather limited and pharmacovigilance does not appear to be high on the political agenda.

Recommendation: Sufficient Financial Means for Relevant Agencies

National and regional competent authorities working under the auspices of national ministries should be endowed with sufficient financial means to fulfil their functions. Likewise, healthcare institutions should be endowed with sufficient means. Sound finances enable healthcare institutions to rely on a stronger workforce which reduces the workload of individual healthcare professionals and increases the possibility of extended reporting of adverse drug reactions.

5.4.3   Perceived Best Practices

However, besides these challenges and the system's shortcomings, the French pharmacovigilance system also exhibits very positive aspects, as discussed below.

Decentralisation

As emphasized by our respondents, one of the major advantages is the decentralised approach to ADR reporting. The close proximity of the 31 regional pharmacovigilance centres situated in hospitals all over the country allows the experts to be close to both healthcare professionals and patients. Moreover, the regional experts are able to keep in contact with both medical and pharmacy students. This profoundly facilitates communication between the relevant reporting and evaluating actors, and the experts remain visible in the healthcare professionals' daily working routine.

Besides collecting and evaluating the reports as well as acting as contact points between reporting actors and the ANSM, the regional centres are also active in research and education. They offer training on pharmacovigilance for healthcare professionals, provide information and expert advice, and serve as the first contact points for patients and practitioners alike. The regional units also provide information on the efficacy and safety of the medicinal products to healthcare professionals and patients.

Furthermore, the reports' assessment and evaluation has been pointed out as advantageous by our interviewees. For each individual case, a causality assessment is conducted. Each report is scientifically evaluated by the regional units before it is forwarded to the ANSM. Thus, low-quality and invalid reports can be largely eliminated before they are entered into the FPD, EMA or WHO databases.

As one of our respondents emphasized, leaving the evaluation to pharmacovigilance experts, usually pharmacists or physicians, was a conscious decision by the relevant actors. Collecting huge amounts of data and leaving signal detection to an algorithm, as for instance in the United Kingdom, was perceived as rather unconstructive.

Awareness Raising

In addition, our respondents identified several good examples regarding education. First, there are some university professors who are specialised in pharmacovigilance. Although they are few, they have a positive influence because they put pharmacovigilance on the agenda of medical faculties and academia. Pharmacovigilance professors enhance the healthcare professionals' knowledge through academic publications, conferences and awareness raising.

Second, a master's programme on pharmacovigilance (cf. Box 5.5) with different specialisations was established by the University of Bordeaux. This programme aims not only at training future professionals in pharmacovigilance and pharmacoepidemiology, but also focuses on establishing an international network of academics and professionals alike which fosters the exchange of knowledge and expertise.

> **Box 5.5**   **Best Practice: Master's Degree in Pharmacovigilance and**
> **Pharmacoepidemiology**
>
> This master's programme is coordinated by the University of Bordeaux and aims at training future professionals in pharmacovigilance as well as fields connected with this issue. Aside from offering basic courses in pharmacovigilance and epidemiology, the programme provides courses in risk identification, pharmacovigilance regulations, public health and risk communication. Moreover, workshops with experts from regulatory agencies and the pharmaceutical industry are held in order to ensure the subjects' practical relevance, as the graduates are expected to work in industry, regulatory bodies and academia alike. Universities from other European countries also participate in this programme to ensure high academic expertise and an international exchange of knowledge.

5.5   ADR Reporting in Portugal

5.5.1   The System

The Portuguese pharmacovigilance system was introduced in 1992. The National Authority of Medicines and Health Products (*Autoridade Nacional do Medicamentos e Produtos de Saúde, I.P.*, or INFARMED) is the country's national competent authority. It supervises and coordinates the regional units and maintains the national ADR database, and is affiliated with the National Health Ministry which is responsible for legislative matters.

The Portuguese pharmacovigilance framework was initially devised as a centralised system, but in the early 2000s turned into a decentralised system (see Duarte et al. 2015; Marques et al. 2015). Today, it is based on four regional pharmacovigilance centres that are in line with Portugal's administrative regions (North, Centre, Lisbon, South). The four regional centres are responsible for collecting, processing and evaluating adverse drug reaction (ADR) reports and maintain their own databases (Mendes et al. 2014).

In doing so, the regional centres collaborate with INFARMED. The Risk Management for Medicines Directorate (*Direção de Gestão do Risco de Medicamentos*) of INFARMED coordinates the national pharmacovigilance database.

There is no separate system for reporting ADRs arising from biological medicines. The Portuguese ADR reporting system is shown in Fig. 5.8.

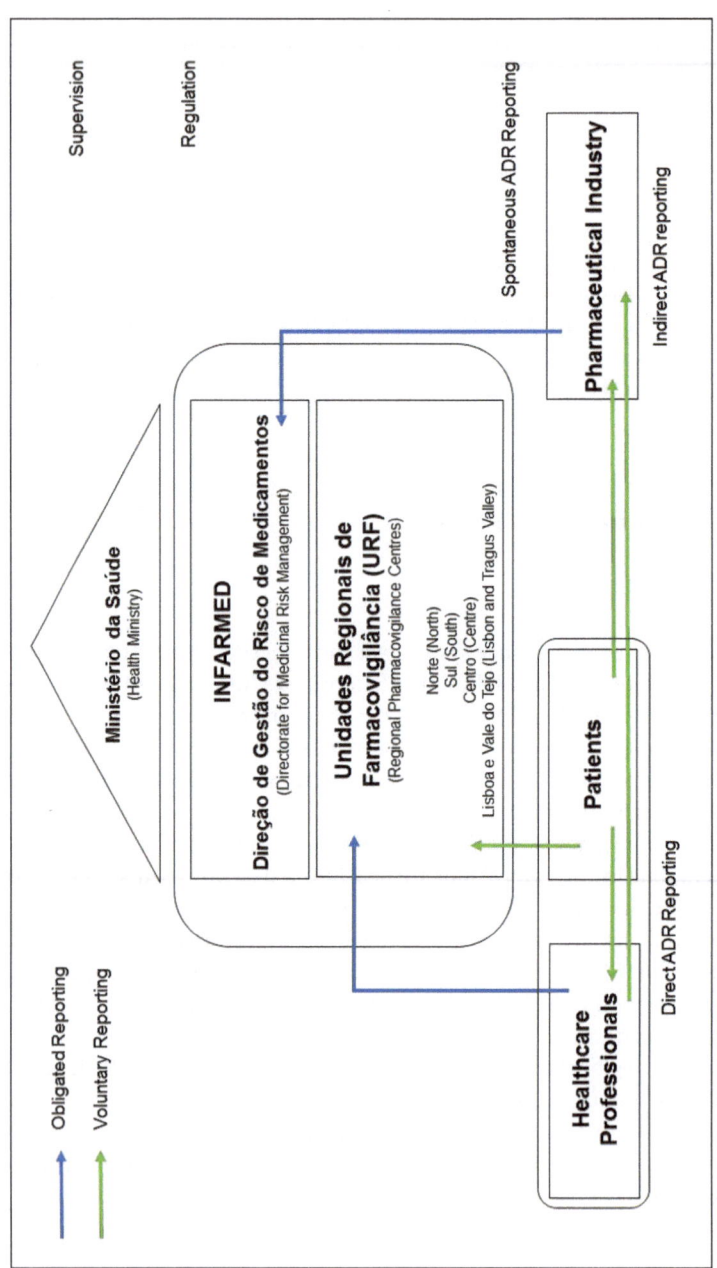

Fig. 5.8   ADR reporting in Portugal (compilation by the authors)

Reporting

In recent years, Portugal has developed a robust pharmacovigilance system, with several actors being allowed to report ADRs (Marques et al. 2016). At the time of system creation in 1992, only physicians were allowed to submit reports. However, pharmacists and nurses were included in 1995 and 1999, respectively. With Directive 2010/84/EU, patients have become the latest addition; today, ADRs can be reported by market authorisation holders, healthcare professionals and patients.

While healthcare professionals and patients submit their reports to the regional pharmacovigilance centres, the respective marketing authorisation holders directly report to the INFARMED sub-unit that is responsible for medicinal risk management.

Reporting by healthcare professionals. All healthcare professionals are legally obligated to report any ADR. Officially, non-compliance is sanctioned. In practice, however, sanctions are not enforced. Healthcare professionals, i.e. physicians, dentists, pharmacists, nurses and medical-technical assistants, are a vital part of the pharmacovigilance system. Depending on their postal code, they have to report adverse reactions to the respective regional centre and need to be available for follow-up questions. A majority of reports is issued by physicians and pharmacists, although some reports are submitted by nurses and medical-laboratory assistants. Healthcare professionals can submit their reports via online forms, e-mail, fax or regular mail.

Reporting by marketing authorisation holders. Marketing authorisation holders are under a legal obligation to report any ADR as well. Yet, while healthcare professionals and patients report to the regional units, the pharmaceutical industry submits its reports directly to INFARMED.

Patient Reporting. Since 2013, patients are also allowed to report suspected ADRs to the regional pharmacovigilance centres. In contrast to professionals and the industry, however, their reports are optional. Reports can be submitted by a number of options, including by telephone, fax, regular mail, e-mail or the online forms provided by the regional centres or INFARMED.

As illustrated by Fig. 5.9, since 2005, marketing authorisation holders submit the majority of reports to INFARMED, followed by physicians and pharmacists. Nurses and patients bring up the rear.

The number of reports has been steadily increasing since the introduction of the system in 1992 (INFARMED 2010). In 2013, the year in which patient reporting was introduced, the number was around 3,400 (Santos n.d.) and in 2014, the number was around 4,600 (Matos et al. 2015). In 2015, the number was around 5,600 (INFARMED 2016). The number of reports submitted by patients, however, is very small, with only 175 reports in 2014 (Santos n.d.). There is also considerable variation in terms of reporting by the regional pharmacovigilance centres (Ribeiro-Vaz et al. 2016).

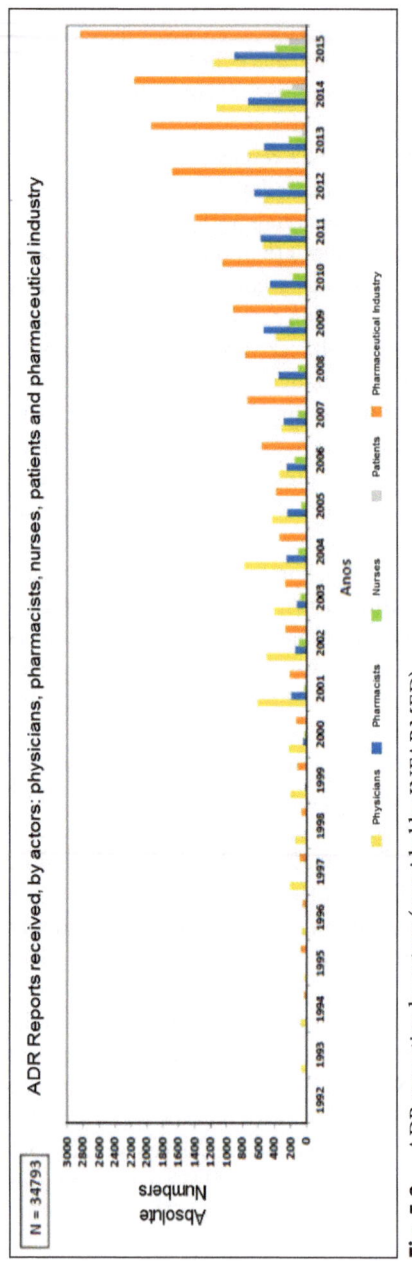

Fig. 5.9   ADR reporting by actors (provided by INFARMED)

Evaluation and Signal Detection

ADR reports submitted by healthcare professionals and patients are collected by the four regional pharmacovigilance centres. The centres receive reports by patients and healthcare professionals assigned by postal code and evaluate them with a team of physicians and pharmacists. Reports submitted by marketing authorisation holders are directly sent to and assessed by INFARMED's Directorate of Risk Management for Medicines.

During the processing of ADR reports, the centres keep in touch with the reporters or directly with the patient, and the necessary information is cross-checked regarding the causality assessment and final review of the adverse reactions. The causality assessment is usually done by clinicians (Inácio et al. 2015). Usually, the regional centres have 30 days from the report's submission for a comprehensive causality assessment before forwarding the report to INFARMED.

Signal detection includes the identification and management of signals and is conducted by the Risk Management for Medicines Directorate of INFARMED. To this end, individual case safety reports (ICSRs), literature and other sources are considered.

In terms of methodology, INFARMED uses multiple approaches, including computerised signal detection methods. However, despite these methods, the assessment of ICSRs remains the most relevant information (INFARMED 2010).

5.5.2 Perceived Challenges

Similar to other countries, underreporting by both healthcare professionals and patients was perceived by our interview partners as a significant shortcoming. The reasons for underreporting are twofold: lack of awareness and time constraints.

Lack of Awareness

First, it has been lamented that the relevant actors are not sufficiently informed that they are able to report. In Portugal, this refers especially to patients. Because patients could only submit reports after Directive 2010/84/EU was transposed into Portuguese legislation in 2013, they are still not yet sufficiently aware of both the possibility to do so and the subject's importance. Despite the fact that patient reporting increased in 2014 and 2015 (cf. Fig. 5.8), indicating that awareness raising is in fact taking place, patients should be more thoroughly informed about the possibility to report ADRs.

Recommendation: Awareness Raising – Patients

In order to tackle underreporting by patients, European, national and regional authorities should invest in awareness-raising campaigns to increase the public knowledge about pharmacovigilance. Even though awareness raising is already taking place in Portugal, efforts in this regard should be enhanced.

However, unawareness is not only a challenge regarding patients, but also regarding healthcare professionals. Here it is important to note that the Portuguese pharmacovigilance system was initiated in the 1990s as a top-down project, and therefore education on this subject is also rather new. Hence, many healthcare professionals are simply not informed about their legal obligation to report every single ADR they encounter.

Moreover, even if healthcare professionals know that they are obligated to report, many physicians and pharmacists are unaware of the importance of reporting all ADRs, and not only new or serious ones. More precisely, while patients are often not aware of the fact that they are able to report, healthcare professionals tend to report only serious or formerly unknown ADRs. Recurrent and non-serious ADRs are largely neglected.

In addition, numerous healthcare professionals do not seem to be aware of the need to report batch numbers in order to ensure the accurate and timely traceability of biological medicines.

All this is especially problematic if the hospital management is also not adequately educated and hence does not consider ADR reporting sufficiently important. Sufficient ADR reporting also depends on the hospital management boards because they can make pharmacovigilance a priority in the working environment and train their medical staff accordingly. However, the management is often perceived as impeding education on the topic and neglecting the issue's importance. Although it is already impeding ADR reporting if practitioners do not consider it relevant, it might be even more dangerous if their superiors label it as insignificant and therefore do not offer practitioners the respective time, information and training they need to report in a responsible manner. This insufficient sense of importance often leads to insufficient prioritisation of the task, which in turn continues to hinder effective ADR reporting in Portugal.

Recommendation: Awareness Raising – Healthcare Professionals

National authorities and healthcare institutions should invest in awareness-raising campaigns to increase professional knowledge about pharmacovigilance and sensitise relevant actors about its particular importance to ensure public health.

In order to improve both the quantity and quality of reports on adverse drug reactions (ADRs), university classes about the importance of pharmacovigilance and the need for ADR reporting should be mandatory for every medical and pharmacy student.

Further, healthcare professionals – including hospital management – should receive additional training to both increase awareness about the particular relevance of ADR reporting related to biologicals and to acquire the necessary skills to ensure the reporting of batch numbers, thereby facilitating the correct and timely traceability of biologicals.

Fear of Litigation

Finally, our interview partners mentioned another issue potentially resulting in the underreporting of ADRs. Even if healthcare professionals are aware of the importance of reporting and have sufficient time to report, they might be unwilling to do so in cases of off-label use. Regardless of the underlying cause of adverse effects, off-label use, medication errors or otherwise, the legal repercussions are a serious concern for healthcare professionals. Hence, it is vital to emphasize that any reporting system should be geared towards the quality of healthcare services and thus be separated from legal proceedings (see EMA 2013). From this perspective, healthcare providers must be assured that ADR reporting has no legal repercussions.

Recommendation: Legal Counselling

The suggested training should include practical and legal counselling in order to alleviate the fear of litigation. While national diversity in health-related and legal terms should be respected, it is important to recognize that fault-based systems are a significant impediment to reporting ADRs. A general and cautious recommendation is to enable healthcare professionals to report ADRs without fear of liability. This could be pursued not only through practical and legal counselling for healthcare professionals, but also by legal means through either strengthening confidentiality or setting up compensation schemes for patients' claims.

Budgetary Constraints

Another challenge pointed out by our respondents is the lack of time to report. This is particularly the case in hospital environments in which physicians and nurses are usually rather overworked. According to our interviewees, adding the comprehensive reporting of every ADR to the usual workload therefore appears to be too challenging. Again, this is a particular obstacle for ADR reporting of biological medicines, the majority of which are dispensed in hospitals.

Thus, there is a perceived shortage of financial and especially human resources which mainly results from lean budgets following the economic crisis in Southern Europe. During the crisis, relevant actors even feared that the pharmacovigilance system could be suspended altogether due to the lack of resources and lack of political priority. The Portuguese pharmacovigilance system is only slowly recovering from the deep financial and personnel cuts in the recent years.

Recommendation: Sufficient Financial Means for Relevant Agencies

National and regional competent authorities working under the auspices of national ministries should be endowed with sufficient financial means to fulfil their functions. Likewise, healthcare institutions should be endowed with sufficient means. Sound finances enable healthcare institutions to rely on a stronger workforce which reduces the workload of individual healthcare professionals and increases the possibility of extended reporting of adverse drug reactions.

5.5.3 Perceived Best Practices

In Portugal's pharmacovigilance system, identified best practices are associated primarily with the four regional pharmacovigilance centres. These best practices concern awareness raising and cooperation.

Awareness Raising

The regional pharmacovigilance centres actively engage in awareness-raising campaigns in order to increase the knowledge and perceived importance of pharmacoyigilance in general and ADR reporting in particular. In order to sensitise these actors about the importance of ADR reporting, regional centres offer internships for pharmacy and medical students, provide lectures and training on pharmacovigilance, and disseminate further relevant information. The southern unit, for instance, educates selected pharmacists on pharmacovigilance and the ADR reporting system.

However, healthcare professionals are not the only target group as many activities are geared towards the general public. One respondent, for instance, mentioned cooperation with public schools aiming to educate both children and their parents.

Cooperation

The aforementioned decentralisation has proven to be vital to strengthen the cooperation of pharmacovigilance centres with universities (Inácio et al. 2015). All regional centres are located within research institutions allowing for close cooperation with the relevant actors in ADR reporting. While the units for Lisbon, South and North are located directly within the universities' medical or pharmacy faculties, the pharmacovigilance unit of the centre region is located within the Association for Innovation and Biomedical Research on Light and Image, a research technology organisation dedicated to the development and clinical research of new products for medicinal therapy and diagnostic imaging.

The regional centres seek to increase the available data on ADRs by collaborating with healthcare organisations. After the initially low number of ADR reports, the northern centre, for instance, established a collaboration protocol with nearby hospitals to collect every suspected case of ADR (Ribeiro-Vaz et al. 2016). This approach requires close collaboration at the personal level between the staff of the pharmacovigilance centre and hospitals. As another instance, respondents identified the collaboration between the southern centre and the rheumatology association. Such close collaboration between the pharmacovigilance centres and other healthcare providers can lead to more and reliable data which considerably facilitates the reports' evaluation and respective signal detection.

Hence, the work by the four regional pharmacovigilance units and especially their strong cooperation with other relevant actors and active engagement in awareness-raising activities has been perceived as particularly conducive to the Portuguese pharmacovigilance system.

5.6   ADR Reporting in Germany

5.6.1   The System

Pharmacovigilance in Germany is based on a highly complex and centralised system that was initiated in the 1970s. Regarding ADR reporting, there are two separate *modus operandi*, depending on whether the product under suspicion is synthetic or biological. Whereas ADRs related to synthetic medicines are centrally collected by the Federal Institute for Drugs and Medical Devices (*Bundesinstitut für Arzneimittel und Medizinprodukte*, or BfArM), ADRs resulting from biologicals must be reported to the Federal Institute for Vaccines (*Paul-Ehrlich-Institut*, or PEI). Even though both agencies are independent and act as centralised agencies, they have a nearly identical legal basis and have similar instruments at their disposal when it comes to pharmacovigilance and ADR reporting (Hagemann and Paeschke 2014).

BfArM and PEI are both under the supervision of the Federal Ministry of Health (Hagemann and Paeschke 2014). Both systems are presented in Fig. 5.10 and 5.11 and are described in the following sections.

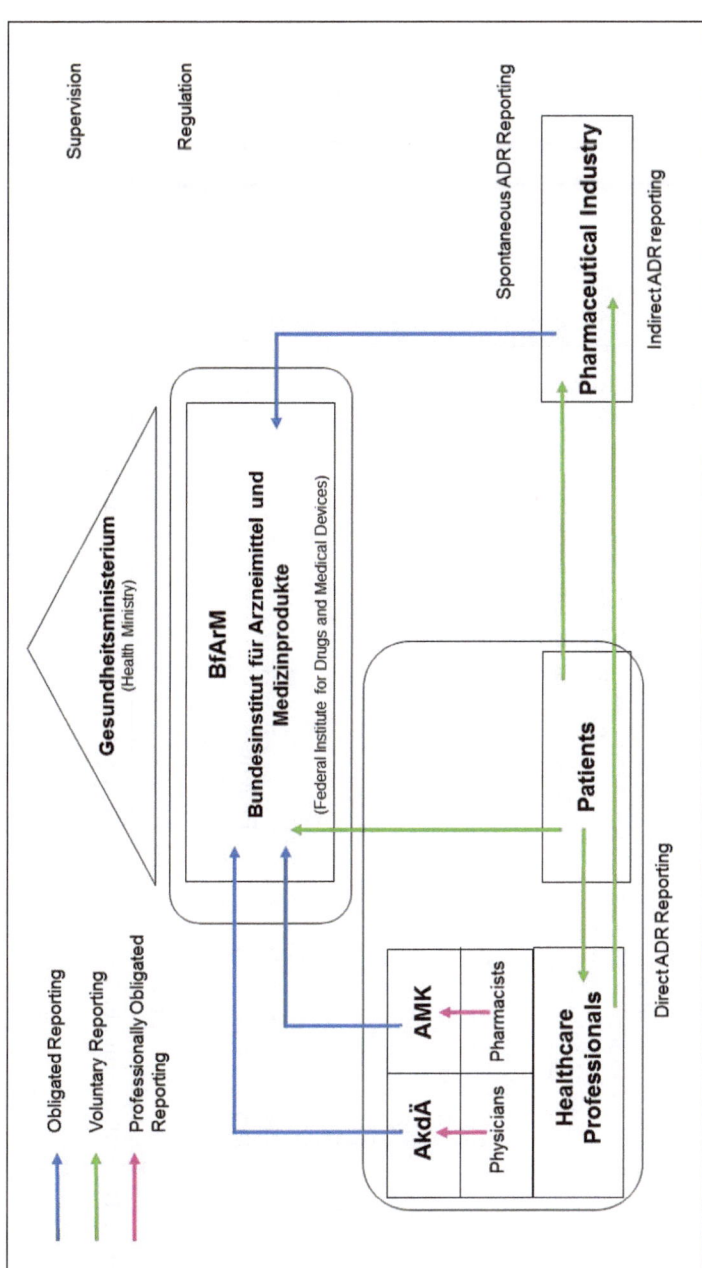

Fig. 5.10 ADR reporting in Germany for synthetic medicines (compilation by the authors)

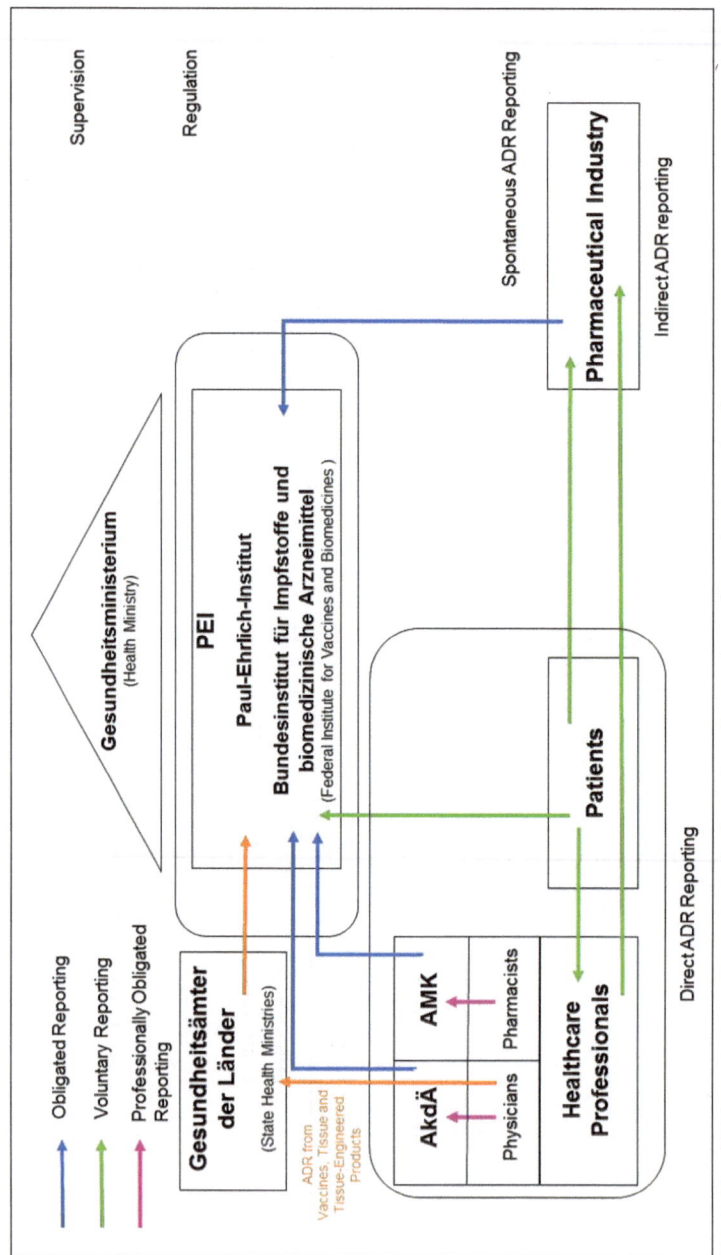

Fig. 5.11 ADR reporting in Germany for biological medicines (compilation by the authors)

Reporting

Healthcare professionals are not legally obligated to report ADRs, neither for synthetic nor biological medicines. They are merely bound by their professional codes of conduct (Ärztliche Berufsordnung, Article 6). Accordingly, there are no sanctions for non-reporting.

Reporting by healthcare professionals. While physicians must report ADRs to the Drug Commission of the German Medical Association (*Arzneikommission der deutschen Ärzteschaft*, or AkdÄ), pharmacists are expected to submit their reports to the largest national association of pharmacists, the Drug Commission of German Pharmacists (*Arzneikommission der Deutschen Apotheker*, or AMK). To facilitate data collection, reports can be submitted online, via regular mail or fax. Physicians and pharmacists receive confirmations of receipt for every submitted report, complemented with additional information and literature regarding the respective ADR. In urgent cases, reporters might be requested to provide further information, such as hospital reports. Sometimes, reporters are contacted via phone for further consultation or follow-up questions in case of lack of clarity.

The physicians' and pharmacists' associations in turn collect, evaluate and – excluding information regarding reporters – forward the reports they receive to BfArM, PEI and marketing authorisation holders. The collaboration between BfArM and the associations is regulated by an agreement created in 1995. Since 2011, there is an additional agreement governing the collaboration with the PEI. Collaboration includes the electronic exchange of ADR reports and reciprocal information exchange regarding newly discovered drug risks. Additionally, the Medical Committee on Drug Safety (**Ärzteausschuss Arzneimittelsicherheit**, or ÄAAS) was initiated at BfArM and PEI, which consists of AkdÄ experts (AkdÄ Tätigkeitsbericht 2015).

Alternatively, healthcare professionals can voluntarily submit reports directly to the respective marketing authorisation holders or the national competent authority BfArM. Submitted reports are disseminated between the different actors so that double reporting is not necessary. In the end, all reports are centrally collected and saved in pseudonomised form by the BfArM, which forwards their reports to the respective marketing authorisation holder and to EMA as well as the WHO.

ADR reporting concerning biologicals works rather similarly. However, instead of reporting to the BfArM, AkdÄ and AKM need to forward the physicians' and pharmacists' reports to the Paul Ehrlich Institute for Vaccines.

However, there is one important difference when it comes to tissues, tissue-engineered products and vaccines. In the case of ADRs related to these products, healthcare professionals do not submit the reports to their respective associations but to the state health authorities (*Gesundheitsämter der Länder*), which carry out a first examination. Subsequently, these health authorities forward the reports to the PEI for central collection.

Reporting by marketing authorisation holders. In contrast to healthcare professionals, marketing authorisation holders are legally obligated to report every case they are informed about to the BfArM or, as regards biologicals, to the PEI (German Drug Law, Chapter 17). In the case of non-compliance, sanctions can be imposed.

Patient Reporting. Patients have various options to report since the transposition of Directive 2010/84/EU in 2012. They can submit reports directly to the national competent authorities, namely the BfArM or the PEI, via phone, e-mail or an online form. Additionally, they can call the respective marketing authorisation holder in order to report an unexpected side effect, or they can consult their physician or pharmacist.

Evaluation and Signal Detection

The evaluation of ADR reports takes place within the AkdÄ and AKM pharmacovigilance units. After the reports' completeness is verified, the reports are scientifically assessed regarding severity, causality and the necessity of further risk-minimising measures, including consultation of a database, medical advisers and research assistants. Evaluation and signal detection is carried out by a software program called ARTEMIS (Adverse Drug Reactions Electronic Management and Information System), which is used to look for similar cases in the shared BfArM and AkdÄ database. In cases of particularly severe ADRs or ambiguous causality assessments, additional scientific statements from experts are collected. Based on these evaluation procedures, selected cases are debated in the respective pharmacovigilance units in order to decide on further procedures. In these settings, relevant public safety issues and necessary measures for risk minimisation – such as additional information for physicians and pharmacists or an alteration of market authorisation – are debated. Relevant safety issues are communicated via the *Deutsches Ärzteblatt,* a weekly magazine, or via drug safety mails (Bronder and Stammschulte 2013).

5.6.2 Perceived Challenges

Even though all respondents considered ADR reporting to work rather efficiently in Germany, several of them emphasized that there are still instances of underreporting, especially by healthcare professionals. As per the interviewees, this can predominantly be attributed to a general lack of awareness and sensitivity regarding ADR reporting as well as insufficient time and personnel.

Lack of Awareness

According to our respondents, the healthcare professionals' lack of awareness regarding ADR reporting can be traced back to various shortcomings in the academic education of the relevant actors. Pharmacovigilance is only included in the curriculum of pharmacy studies, while other medical curricula do not impart any knowledge on drug safety in general and on pharmacovigilance in particular.

Recommendation: Awareness Raising – Healthcare Professionals

In order to tackle underreporting by healthcare providers, national authorities and healthcare institutions should invest in awareness-raising campaigns to increase professional knowledge about pharmacovigilance and sensitise relevant actors about its particular importance to ensure public health.

To improve both the quantity and quality of ADR reports, university classes about the importance of pharmacovigilance and ADR reporting should be mandatory for every medical and pharmacy student.

In addition, European, national or regional authorities should organise advanced post-graduate training on a regular basis to ensure that healthcare professionals acquire the necessary skills to cope with the complex task of ADR reporting.

It was further indicated that patients are not sufficiently aware that they are able to report and do not know how to do so. This suggests that the quantity of ADR reports could be increased if patients were better informed. Additionally, respondents pointed out that reporting mechanisms for patients were still rather complex.

In addition, the quality of submitted ADR reports has been criticized by several interview partners. More precisely, it was pointed out that reports submitted via the national competent authority's online forms are frequently incomplete. This leads to severe problems for data evaluation and signal detection. Incomplete reports cannot be processed adequately and are therefore invalid. Accordingly, missing information needs to be gathered in a follow-up process and this means a considerable increase in workload for the relevant actors.

In line with this, our respondents generally suggested that direct patient reporting was rather unconstructive. Instead, they agreed that patients who suspect an ADR should consult their physician first and file their reports in collaboration with them.

> **Recommendation: Awareness Raising – Patients**
>
> In order to tackle underreporting by patients, European, national and regional authorities should invest in awareness-raising campaigns to increase the public knowledge about pharmacovigilance.
>
> Authorities should raise awareness in the short term through various means of communication (e.g. websites, social media, leaflets) as well as in the long term through cooperation with schools to educate future generations.
>
> In order to facilitate ADR reporting by patients, Member States should offer a wide range of possible communication channels, including web-based and paper-based formats. Both web-based and paper-based formats should be designed to be as user-friendly as possible. For web-based formats, IT solutions should be developed to guide patients through the format and to ensure the completeness of reports. All formats should be accompanied by accessible manuals written in layman's terms.

A first step in this direction is indicated by ongoing discussions about introducing a smartphone app intending to render ADR reporting more accessible to the public and thereby reduce reporting hurdles for patients. We consider this a good approach which should be pursued further.

Lack of Interconnectivity

Moreover, some respondents pointed out that the IT infrastructure of hospitals, pharmacies, associations and institutes is by no means connected. In some cases, there is still the need to manually transfer data from one system to another. This is a very time-consuming, complex and resource-intensive process, which is prone to mistakes and transcription errors.

A closely related problem is the duplication of ADR reports that occurs when identical reports are submitted by different actors, e.g. when patients report ADRs directly to the national competent authority and subsequently consult healthcare professionals, who then report the incident to the national competent authority a second time. Due to the particularly restrictive data protection laws in Germany, it is practically impossible to identify these duplications. In addition, unique characteristics are omitted from the reports at a very early stage of the process. Even though this ensures proper data protection, at the same time the detection of duplications is rendered impossible.

Recommendation: Harmonisation of IT Systems

In order to cope with information overload and to facilitate the process of submitting ADR reports, national and regional competent authorities should improve interconnectivity of IT systems, as for instance those of general practitioners, hospitals, pharmacies and the ADR reporting system.

In addition, the process of "who reports to whom" could be further facilitated and clarified, allowing for a more streamlined process and less data duplication.

Budgetary Constraints

Several interviewees described challenges regarding financial resources. Both national competent authorities, i.e. BfArM and PEI, are financially dependent on the Federal Ministry of Health. Accordingly, there is no room for quick and independent decision-making, resulting in delayed and insufficient reactions to changing demands.

Recommendation: Sufficient Financial Means for Relevant Actors

National and regional competent authorities working under the auspices of national ministries should be endowed with sufficient financial means to fulfil their functions. Likewise, healthcare institutions should be endowed with sufficient means. Sound finances enable healthcare institutions to rely on a stronger workforce which reduces the workload of individual healthcare professionals and increases the possibility of extended reporting of ADRs.

Incomplete Reports

Finally, our respondents are largely satisfied with the functioning of ADR reporting and the identification and traceability of biologicals. The only caveat identified is that the product name and batch number cannot be reported in all cases. *Inter alia*, this can be attributed to rather vague legal requirements. However, the currently discussed Fourth Amendment to the German Drug Law (*4. Gesetz zur Änderung arzneimittelrechtlicher und anderer Vorschriften*) requires that both the brand name and batch number must be reported for ADRs relating to biologicals, which is a step in the right direction.

5.6.3   Perceived Best Practices

The German pharmacovigilance system is deeply entrenched and well-appointed with manifold experts in the field. Because the pharmacovigilance system has been in place for more than 40 years, experience and routine both contribute to effective ADR reporting. Moreover, identification and traceability of biological medicines works particularly well because there is a separate system for biologicals.

Even though the German pharmacovigilance system is centralised, the national competent authorities are usually not directly contacted by healthcare professionals. Instead the physicians' and pharmacists' associations collect the reports and subsequently forward them. Hence, these associations act as points of contact between reporters and the authorities, thereby assuming a mediating role and allow for better communication between the relevant actors.

Awareness Raising

The national competent authorities provide several possibilities for engagement and educational activities for actors in the pharmacovigilance system. Healthcare professionals, patients and pharmaceutical companies can contact the authorities at any time in order to receive additional information on certain products or ADR reporting.

Additionally, Germany established several systems for spreading new information on risks of medicinal products to healthcare professionals. The so-called red-hand letter (*Rote-Hand-Brief*) is distributed via regular mail. The red hand printed on the cover signals that the letter does not contain an advertisement but important information related to pharmacovigilance (for further information see cf. Box 5.6).

Further, since December 2016, the so-called blue-hand letter (*Blaue-Hand-Brief*) has been introduced. Blue-hand letters contain additional and relevant educational information and material on specific medicines (cf. Box 5.6)

Additionally, the AMK established, together with the Confederation of the Pharmaceutical Wholesale Trade (PHAGRO), an efficient fax information system aiming to inform pharmacists and other healthcare professionals about urgent risks (cf. Box 5.7).

Cooperation

Pharmacovigilance educational and research centres are important for improving ADR reporting. A particularly good example in Germany is the Institute for Clinical Teratology and Drug Risk Assessment in the Pregnancy and Nursing Period (*Pharmakovigilanzzentrum Embryonaltoxikologie,* or Embryotox), which is located in the Charité hospital in Berlin. This institute serves as a consultancy centre for healthcare professionals working in hospitals and advises the national competent authorities whenever problems or questions referring to ADRs in pregnancy and nursing periods arise. It also maintains an online database which is accessible to everyone.[6] Moreover, it can forward ADRs to the national competent authorities.

Another advisory body in the German pharmacovigilance system is the Medical Committee on Drug Safety (ÄAAS), which also advises the national competent authorities with expertise on specific risks of medicinal products.

Box 5.6   Red- and blue-hand letters

In 1969, the German Pharmaceutical Industry Association introduced the red hand as a symbol to indicate the importance of the information provided in the letter. These letters with the red hand are distributed to all healthcare professionals. The unique red hand logo signals that the letter does not contain an advertisement but important information on newly detected risks of medicines or a defective batch. The red-hand letters are distributed in consultation with BfArM and PEI and are a common way to communicate medicinal risks in Germany.

The newly introduced blue-hand letter (in December 2016) contains educational material that has been approved by BfArM and PEI. More precisely, the letters provide additional information complementing the package leaflets and the summary of product characteristics and are directed to physicians, pharmacists or patients in order to alert them about certain risks. It is expected that the blue-hand letters will contribute towards improving the safe and correct use of medicinal products.

---

6   www.embryotox.de.

Box 5.7   AMK/PHAGRO Schnellinformationssystem

Moreover, the AMK, in collaboration with the association of pharmaceutical wholesaler trading companies (PHAGRO), distributes information to pharmacies via a fax information system (*AMK/PHAGRO Schnellinformationssystem*). This system was established in 1996 aiming at providing important and urgent information on drug safety risks on short notice. In the case of an emergency, the AMK, in close cooperation with the marketing authorization holder and the responsible national competent authority, drafts an informational notice, which includes the medicine's name, the batch number and a description of the potential dangers. Moreover, recommended actions are enclosed. The informational notice is distributed via fax to every wholesale trader in Germany; these traders print them and enclose them with the invoices and delivery notes accompanying every single shipment to pharmacies. Because pharmacies are usually supplied every day, the informational notices reach end consumers very quickly.

An additional e-mail and fax system sends the information notices to the AkdÄ, hospital pharmacies, the German army medical service, public institutes, and diverse competent authorities at the state and federal levels. In addition, the informational notice is published, often including additional information, in the next AMK newsletter.

References

ANSM (2016). *Annual Report 2015*. Last accessed on 04.11.2016: ansm.sante.fr/content/download/97375/1237039/.../ANSM-RA-*15*_EN_oct2016.pdf

AkdÄ (2016). *Tätigkeitsbericht 2015*. Last accessed on 02.12.2016: www.akdae.de/Kommission/Organisation/Aufgaben/Taetigkeitsbericht.pdf

Bronder, E., Stammschulte, T. (2013). *Nebenwirkungen von Arzneimitteln: Meldung an die Arzneimittelkommission der deutschen Ärzteschaft, Erfassung in einer Datenbank und Bewertung.* Ärzteblatt Thüringen, Ausgabe 12/2013: 670-672.

Caron, J., Gautier, S., Mallaret, M. (2014). Spontaneous Reporting: France. Andrews, E., Moore, N. (eds) (2014). *Mann's Pharmacovigilance*. Wiley-Blackwell.

Casassus, B. (2016). *Drug Scandals in France: Have the Lessons Been Learnt?* The Lancet 2016/388: 550-552.

Duarte, M., Ferreira, P., Soares, M., Cavaco, A., Martins, A. P. (2015). *Community Pharmacists' Attitudes towards Adverse Drug Reaction Reporting and their Knowledge of the New Pharmacovigilance Legislation in the Southern Region of Portugal: A Mixed Methods Study*. Drugs and Therapy Perspectives 31 (9): 316-322.

EMA (2013). *Medication Errors Workshop – Workshop Report*. EMA/144458/2013 Patient Health Protection 06.05.2013.

Fimea (2010). Guideline 2/2010 – Reporting of Adverse Drug Reactions. Last accessed on 22.05.2016: https://www.fimea.fi/documents/542809/844142/17296_Ohje_2_2010_Haittavaikutusten_ilmoittaminen_EN.pdf.

Fimea Administrative Guidelines 2/2013 (2013). *Reporting of Adverse Drug Reactions, 3428/03.01.01/2012*. Last accessed on 22.05.2016: https://www.fimea.fi/.../23514_Ohje_2_2013_EN.pdf

Finnish Communicable Diseases Act (583/1986). Last accessed on 22.05.2016: www.finlex.fi/fi/laki/kaannokset/1986/en19860583.pdf

Foy, M. (2015). *eHealth – The Road towards More Efficient and Integrated Care Solutions for Patients*. Presentation for MHRA.

Hagemann, U., Paeschke, N. (2014). How Pharmacovigilance Is Organised in Germany. In: Andrews, E., Moore, N. (eds) (2014). *Mann's Pharmacovigilance*. Wiley-Blackwell Oxford.

Inácio, P., Airaksinen, M., Cavaco, A. (2015). Language Does Not Come "in Boxes": Assessing Discrepancies between Adverse Drug Reactions Spontaneous Reporting and MedDRA® Codes in European Portuguese. Research in Social and Administrative Pharmacy 11: 664-674.

INFARMED (2011). *Boletim de Farmacovigilância*. Boletim de Farmacovigilância 15 (2).

INFARMED (2016). *Boletim de Farmacovigilância*. Boletim de Farmacovigilância 20 (2).

Marques, J. I. O., Polonia, J. M. J., Figueiras, A. G., Santos, C. M., Herdeiro, M. F. (2016). *Nurses' Attitudes and Spontaneous Adverse Drug Reaction Reporting: A Case-Control Study in Portugal*. Journal of Nursing Management 24: 409-416.

Matos, C., Van Hunsel, F., Joaquim, J. (2015). *Are Consumers Ready to Take Part in the Pharmacovigilance System? A Portuguese Preliminary Study Concerning ADR Reporting*. European Journal of Clinical Pharmacology 71: 883-890.

Mendes, D., Alves, C., Batel-Marques, F. (2014). *Safety Profiles of Adalimumab, Etanercept and Infliximab: A Pharmacovigilance Study Using a Measure of Disproportionality in a Database of Spontaneously Reported Adverse Events*. Journal of Clinical Pharmacy and Therapeutics 39: 307-313.

MHRA (2016). *Guidance on Adverse Drug Reactions*. Last accessed on 13.09.2016: https://www.gov.uk/government/uploads/system/uploads/attachment_data/file/403098/Guidance_on_adverse_drug_reactions.pdf

Mullard, A. (2011). *Mediator Scandal Rocks French Medical Community*. The Lancet 2011/377: 890-892.

Ribeiro-Vaz, I., Santos, C., Cruz-Correira, R. (2016). Promoting Adverse Drug Reaction Reporting: Comparison of Different Approaches. Revista Saúde Pública 50 (14): 1-9.

Santos, A. (n.d.). *Direct Patient Reporting in the European Union: A Snapshot of Reporting Systems in Seven Member States*. Health Action International. Last accessed on 02.12.2016: http://haiweb.org/publication/direct-patient-reporting-in-the-eu-a-snapshot-of-reporting-systems-in-seven-member-states/

THL (2016). *National Institute for Health and Welfare – Vaccinations*. Last accessed on 04.10.2016: https://www.thl.fi/fi/web/thlfi-en/statistics/information-on-statistics/quality-descriptions/vaccinations

URPL (2015). Jak zgłaszać działania niepożądane (How to Report Side Effects). On Youtube posted by URPLWMiPB on 10.02.2015. Last accessed on 25.09.2016: https://www.youtube.com/watch?v=mE_EbeE7ado&feature=youtu.be

URPL (2014). Zgłaszanie działań niepożądanych (Reporting Adverse Events). On Youtube posted by URPLWMiPB on 14.02.2014. Last accessed on 25.09.2016: https://www.youtube.com/watch?v=g2H8BOq0UOc

Yellow Card Centre Wales (n.d.). *Annual Report Year 2013-2014.* Last accessed 13.09.2016: http://www.yellowcardwales.org/pdfs/YCCW%20Annual%20Report%202013-14-%20 Final.pdf

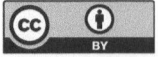

Challenges and Best Practices in Perspective

6

In this chapter, we compare the challenges and best practices identified in the country chapters so that the in-depth analysis of selected Member States is complemented with a broader overview. In doing so, we aim to provide a better understanding of the practical implementation of the new European Union (EU) pharmacovigilance legislation across Member States.

The chapter is structured as follows. First, the national pharmacovigilance systems are compared regarding their structural factors as well as their institutional frameworks. The second section deals with the main finding of this study, namely the underreporting of adverse drug reactions (ADRs) in the Member States. This finding is substantiated by identifying problems in terms of batch numbers for biological medicinal products (biologicals), scientific evaluation, signal detection and information processing. Finally, we present a comparison of factors contributing to underreporting. The key factors in this respect are as follows:

- Lack of awareness
- Complexity of ADR reporting
- Lack of cooperation
- Interconnectivity problems

Key factors and the underlying reasons have been discovered through repeated rounds of trial and error, relying on pharmacovigilance literature, reports on the effectiveness of pharmacovigilance systems and interview data gathered for the selected cases. By probing the empirical evidence with a variety of categorisations, we aimed to find the right balance in the accurate reporting of specific reasons while relying on key factors for meaningful comparative analysis and generalisation.

6.1   Pharmacovigilance Systems

The objective of this section is to provide a comparative overview of the national pharmacovigilance systems. As indicated in Chapter 3, EU pharmacovigilance is a multi-level system where actors are linked through multiple inter-institutional relations. Adding to this complexity, national pharmacovigilance systems themselves comprise a multitude of actors, which cooperate in line with patterns of implementation (see Chapter 5).

Level of Centralisation

Due to different healthcare policies and institutions, there is considerable variation in the level of centralisation. Whereas some Member States have centralised systems of pharmacovigilance, others have decentralised systems. Germany, the United Kingdom, Finland and Poland have centralised systems; Portugal and France have decentralised systems. The decentralised systems are characterised by having regional centres for collecting and processing pharmacovigilance data.

The level of centralisation, however, is not set in stone. Whereas Portugal has moved from a centralised system to a decentralised system in the early 2000s, the United Kingdom has set up regional Yellow Card centres.

Although the system in Germany is centralised, sectoral associations of physicians and pharmacists provide functional links between patients, healthcare providers and national competent authorities. Hence, the system can be characterised as highly complex. Depending on the type of medicine, two different national agencies are at the centre of ADR reporting.

Supervision

In terms of supervision, the national agencies implementing pharmacovigilance are usually supervised by the health and social security ministries. In implementing pharmacovigilance, the agencies are also accountable to respective ministries. In the sample, however, Finland and Poland are exceptions. Even though Fimea and URPL are officially headed by ministries that set the legal guidelines, they are *de facto* independent and do not have to justify their decisions.

Separate Systems for Biologicals

There is considerable variation among Member States regarding the classification of biologicals. Whereas some Member States operate separate systems for biologicals, others treat biologicals as part of their general pharmacovigilance systems. In the sample, only Germany operates a separate system for biologicals. In line with its complex system, there are two national agencies operating in Germany, one dealing with synthetic medicines and the other one with biologicals. Finland and Poland have a system for biological vaccines. However, Portugal, France and the United Kingdom have no separate system.[7]

This variation is not surprising, given the fact that there is no unambiguous agreement among Member States about how to classify biologicals (see Klein et al. 2015).

Legal Requirements

In the sample, almost all Member States have legal requirements for healthcare professionals to report ADRs, i.e. Portugal, France, Finland and Poland. In France, this includes brand names and batch numbers of biologicals (Vermeer et al. 2015: 8). In Germany and the United Kingdom, there are no legal requirements in place, and hence ADR reporting in these countries is based on professional obligations and codes of conduct. In Poland, there are legal requirements but no punishment in the case of non-compliance.

Patients are generally not required to report ADRs, in contrast to marketing authorisation holders that are legally obligated to report them in all countries under investigation.

Prescribing Medicines

There is also considerable variation among Member States regarding the practice of prescribing medicines. In line with the different national health systems, doctors and pharmacists might substitute different medicines with the same active substance. Previous studies have shown that prescribers often communicate only the international non-proprietary name (INN) in ADR reporting (Dolinar and Reilly 2014). Merely indicating the INN in an ADR report can be misleading, though, as two different medicines (the original biological and the new biosimilar) may have the same non-proprietary scientific name. However, while some stakeholders call for a change to such practices, the majority of Member States maintain that biosimilars and reference products should be closely aligned and that using different INNs undermines such an alignment (see European Commission Pharmaceutical Committee 2013).

---

7   Despite the absence of a separate system, biologicals receive particular attention in the United Kingdom. Biologicals are discussed by MHRA experts in separate meetings.

Tab. 6.1 Comparison of the national pharmacovigilance systems (compilation by the authors)

	United Kingdom	Finland	Poland	France	Portugal	Germany
Established	1964	1982	1971	1973	1992	1970s
System	Centralised	Centralised	Centralised	Decentralised	Decentralised	Centralised
Separate system for biologicals	No	Only for vaccines	Only for vaccines	No	No	Yes
Supervision	Department of Health	Ministry of Social Affairs and Welfare	Health Ministry	Ministry for Health and Social Security	National Health Ministry	Federal Ministry of Health
National Competent Authority	MHRA	Fimea	URPL	ANSM	INFARMED	BfArM and PEI
Reporting – Healthcare Professionals	Professionally obliged. Report via YCS system to MHRA.	Only obligated in case of vaccines. Report synthetic products to Fimea and vaccines to THL.	Legally obligated. Report to URPL.	Legally obligated. Report to ANSM's regional units.	Legally obligated. Report to INFARMED's regional units.	Professionally obligated. Report to AkdÄ or AKM which forward reports for synthetic products to BfArM and for biologicals to PEI. Report vaccines to state health authorities.
Reporting – Patients	Voluntary. Since 2005. Report to HCPs, MAHs or via YCS system to MHRA.	Voluntary. Since 2012. Report to HCPs, MAHs or Fimea.	Voluntary. Since 2012. Report to HCPs, MAHs or URPL.	Voluntary. Since 2011. Report to HCPs, MAHs, ANSM or regional units.	Voluntary. Since 2013. Report to HCPs, MAHs, IN-FARMED or regional units.	Voluntary. Since 2012. Report to HCPs, MAHs, or BfArM/PEI.
Reporting – Marketing Authorisation Holders	Legally obligated. Report to MHRA database.	Legally obligated. Report to Fimea.	Legally obligated. Report to URPL.	Legally obligated. Report to ANSM.	Legally obligated. Report to IN-FARMED.	Legally obligated. Report to BfArM or PEI.
Evaluation and Signal Detection	No evaluation. Signal detection by MHRA.	Fimea	URPL	Regional units	Regional units	AkdÄ, AKM, BfArM and PEI

6.2   Major Challenges

The objective of this section is to present underreporting as the main finding of this study.

Underreporting

The most important challenge for the effective implementation of Directive 2010/84/EU is the underreporting of ADRs. In all Member States in the sample, respondents highlight this (the United Kingdom, Poland, France, Portugal and Germany). This study thereby confirms previous studies based on the comparative analysis of cases selected on their variation in terms of national health systems.

This is remarkable, given that in 22 countries (79 percent) reporting of ADRs is a legal obligation for healthcare professionals, and the percentage of countries with mandatory reporting of ADRs for vaccines is even higher, i.e. 26 countries (89 percent) (Šarinić et al. 2016).

The highest percentage (38 percent) of all ADR reports is received via web-based applications, even though the number of Member States having web-based reporting is lower than the number of Member States with mail-reporting channels available (21 vs. 28, respectively) (Šarinić et al. 2016). In our sample, only a minority of the French regional pharmacovigilance centres appeared to have websites and thereby web-based reporting formats. In Finland, even though online reporting is possible for physicians and pharmacists, patients have to resort to regular mail. All Member States have ADR reporting forms available on their national competent authorities' websites (SCOPE).

There are two important aspects to underreporting: the quantity and quality of information. Quantity refers to the number of ADR reports; quality refers to the value of information. Both dimensions are sometimes mutually exclusive, as increases in quantity might lead to decreases in quality. Whereas quantity of information is important, an appropriate level of quality is essential for effective pharmacovigilance. Some respondents fret about incomplete reports, requiring follow-up and thereby further increasing the workload (Germany). Other respondents were rather satisfied with the quality of ADR reports but criticized the number of reports submitted (Poland).

Information Overload

Furthermore, information overload can make it difficult to detect signals (Germany). This problem is exacerbated by the fact that the legislation allows the collection of information from all possible and available sources such as patients and literature reports. This also leads to an increased pool of information from which relevant signals can be analysed (Borg et al. 2015: 121).

There is considerable variation in the Member States regarding evaluation and signal detection.

In the United Kingdom, there is no evaluation of reports before signal detection; due to the large quantity of information, signal detection has been automated. After prioritising detected signals, the national competent authority, the Medicines and Healthcare Products Regulatory Agency (MHRA), forwards serious cases to EMA.

Causality Assessments

In the two decentralised systems, Portugal and France, ADR reports are collected and evaluated by the regional units. However, problems in terms of quantity and quality might lead to problems in terms of causality assessments (France). After the evaluation, including the causality assessment, the reports are forwarded to the national competent authorities. Reports by marketing authorisation holders are forwarded directly to the national agencies.

Traceability of Biologicals

Previous studies showed that the reporting of batch numbers and traceability of biologicals is subject to considerable variation among Member States (Vermeer et al. 2015; see also European Commission 2015). Various studies on ADR reporting revealed that batch numbers were available for only a limited number of suspected biologicals (Vermeer et al. 2013: 620-621; see also Vermeer et al. 2015: 6).

Again, this study substantiates this. Respondents in various Member States in the sample confirm that reporting batch numbers remains a challenge (the United Kingdom). Batch numbers are reported infrequently (France) or not at all (Poland). Only in Finland did the reporting of batch numbers satisfy the respondents which has been corroborated by Fimea's statistics.

Strengthening Patient Involvement

One of the aims of Directive 2010/84/EU is to strengthen patient involvement in the safety monitoring of medicines. All 28 Member States have patient reporting systems in place, with the majority initiating them in 2012-2013 (although the first Member States to introduce this process did so only starting in 1968 and the second time in 1996). Overall, the number of individual patient reports from the European Economic Area has increased over the two and a half years of the reporting period by around 50 percent. This includes ADR reports not submitted by other reporters such as healthcare professionals, which represent information that would not otherwise be captured (Commission 2016).

However, reporting ADRs regarding biologicals and respective traceability remains a challenge when it comes to patient reporting. For instance, batch numbers have to be displayed on each package in the United Kingdom, but patients often do not have access to the package when the drug is administered in a hospital setting.

6.3 Comparison of Factors Contributing to Underreporting

The objective of this section is to compare factors contributing to underreporting and thereby to put into comparative perspective the challenges and best practices in national pharmacovigilance systems.

6.3.1 Lack of Awareness

As described above, awareness as an analytical category for comparison includes a number of factors, such as not only the general awareness of the obligation to report, but also indifference regarding the importance of ADR reporting.

Member States have focused on informing healthcare professionals and patients about the importance of ADR reporting, particularly regarding biologicals (see Vermeer et al. 2015). The importance of raising awareness has been emphasized as part of the SCOPE implementation project (Jadeja and Barrow 2016: 59).

However, the study reveals that lack of awareness is a prevalent feature in all the Member States of our sample (the United Kingdom, Finland, Poland, France, Portugal and Germany). Yet lacking awareness concerns healthcare professionals and patients in varying degrees. Whereas in Finland, most healthcare professionals are aware of their obligation to report ADRs, the level of public awareness is particularly low. Similarly, in the United Kingdom about 80 percent of healthcare professionals know about the Yellow Card Scheme, while only 10 percent of patients had heard about this.

Lack of Awareness Regarding Biologicals

In some Member States, lack of awareness regarding biologicals seems to be particularly severe (Poland, Portugal). This is an interesting finding because Portugal's decentralised system seems well-equipped regarding a key recommendation about the role of regional pharmacovigilance centres for awareness-raising campaigns (Jadeja and Barrow 2016: 59-60). Also, Poland revealed that problems regarding ADR reporting of biologicals mainly stemmed from its inexperience and thus its unawareness in the field.

Legal Framework

As explained in the fundamentals regarding pharmacovigilance (see Chapter 2), legal ramifications of ADR reporting due to liability claims is a specific factor of awareness. While healthcare professionals are bound by the legal systems in which they operate, awareness regarding the legal ramifications and how they affect ADR reporting is a key recommendation (see Chapter 7).

In general, the possibility of liability claims presents an important impediment for ADR reporting. The SCOPE data demonstrates that the quantity can be enhanced by exempting healthcare professionals from liability when they report ADRs that possibly resulted from medication errors (Šarinić et al. 2016: 218). In this context, our study reveals that liability claims are feared by healthcare professionals in Poland, France and Portugal, which impedes ADR reporting in these countries.

In a similar vein, ADRs and the reporting thereof are sometimes perceived as a failure of healthcare professionals associated with a threat to professional reputation.

6.3.2   Complexity of ADR Reporting

Complexity as an analytical category encompasses a number of factors related to the task of ADR reporting, including not only reporting logistics, but also constraints in the work environment of healthcare professionals.

In our study, factors impeding ADR reporting due to complexity have been frequently highlighted by respondents and it appears that such complexity affects both the quantity and quality of ADR reporting.

For instance, in Finland only healthcare professionals (physicians and pharmacists) are able to report online, while patients and nurses have to report through regular mail. In Germany, duplications are difficult to filter out because strict data protection laws make it difficult to connect databases.

SCOPE data reveals that offering background and supplementary information within the electronic or the paper version of the reporting form enhances the quality of the submitted reports (Jan and Radecka 2015: 63-64). However, a number of respondents, especially in Poland, France and Portugal, cite high workload as an impediment to more effective pharmacovigilance.

ADR reporting is also perceived as time-consuming and complex (France, Portugal). The necessity of having to be available for follow-up questions further disincentives healthcare professionals, given that reporting is not a one-off activity, but may turn into a lengthy process. This also has negative consequences for data quantity.

Training in Pharmacovigilance

The lack of quality (and also underreporting and the lack of quantity) are related to the neglect of pharmacovigilance training during medical and pharmaceutical education. This is the case in the United Kingdom and Germany. Finland, however, offers a very elaborate educational system for healthcare professionals regarding pharmacovigilance, and France is one of the first Member States to introduce a master's programme in pharmacovigilance.

The SCOPE data shows that only a minority of the national competent authorities (e.g. the MHRA) offer e-learning tools and online educational materials for healthcare professionals, although these tools are very efficient and considerably improve professional training (Jadeja and Barrow 2016: 57). Yet in order to implement legal provisions of EU pharmacovigilance to full effect, training is essential for internalising practices that are conducive to the realisation of these provisions. Because most ADRs are well-known effects of old drugs, harm might be avoided if healthcare professionals (and also patients) were better trained or at least informed (Moore and Begaud 2010).

In general, national pharmacovigilance systems must be seen as dependent on general policy developments. In the current political climate, one such development is the structural scarcity of funding for regulatory activity.

Financial Resources

Pharmacovigilance is no exception here, with several Member States in the sample having to fulfil their functions with limited financial resources (e.g. France, Germany). While scarce finances are an issue across the board, the problem is acute in Southern European Member States such as Portugal that were particularly affected by the economic crisis.

6.3.3 Lack of Cooperation

Cooperation is an essential analytical category for contextualising individual ADR reporting by healthcare professionals in complex national systems of pharmacovigilance.

A multitude of actors in national pharmacovigilance systems require cooperation among pharmacovigilance-related institutions in order to ensure system effectiveness. The SCOPE authors recommend fostering the exchange of information and the sharing of best practices among the Member States and the relevant stakeholders (Jadeja and Barrow 2016: 58). Aside from interconnecting state authorities, the SCOPE authors also suggest enhancing collaboration with patient organisations and professional associations on a national as well as an international level (Jadeja and Barrow 2016: 58).

However, there is considerable variation in the Member States due to their institutional differences. At one end of the spectrum is Portugal with the successful cooperation of agencies, healthcare professionals and universities. At the other end of the spectrum is Poland with no cooperation between relevant actors.

6.3.4   Interconnectivity Problems

Due to the increase of ADR reporting since the adoption of Directive 2010/84/EU, the technical infrastructure for data processing and interconnectivity of databanks is a particular challenge. In order to cope with increasing data, Member States have introduced new functionalities to reporting systems and cooperation between hospital and pharmacy IT systems (Vermeer et al. 2015: 8).

SCOPE data suggests that sound and uniform IT systems for reporting ADRs on a national as well as an international level would lead to increased efficiency, better data quality and error prevention (Šarinić et al. 2016: 220).

However, the case studies highlight specific problems in terms of interconnectivity. Our study shows that different IT systems and separated online portals are seen as impeding interconnectivity in a number of Member States (the United Kingdom, France and Germany).

In conclusion, it is important to emphasize that healthcare policies of Member States differ considerably. Accordingly, a comparison of challenges and best practices can inform mutual learning, yet such learning is contingent on deep-seated structural and cultural factors that affect the national implementation of EU pharmacovigilance legislation.

Furthermore, broader policy developments have significant effects on the implementation of pharmacovigilance. For instance, due to strict data protection laws, Germany can be characterised as a laggard in pharmacovigilance research (see Douros et al. 2016). Due to the Mediator scandal, France has to be mentioned as well, given that the national pharmacovigilance system is still impeded by systematic difficulties.

In the final chapter, we suggest several recommendations aiming to cope with these persistent challenges in national ADR reporting systems and thereby to improve the practical implementation of Directive 2010/84/EU.

References

Borg et al. (2015). *European Union Pharmacovigilance Capabilities: Potential for the New Legislation*. Ther Adv Drug Safety 6 (4): 120-140.

Dolinar, R., Reilly, M. (2014). *Biosimilars Naming, Label Transparency and Authority of Choice – Survey Findings among European Physicians*. Generics and Biosimilars Initiative 3 (2): 58-62.

Douros, A. et al. (2016). *Pharmakovigilanz in Deutschland*. Internist 57: 616-623.

European Commission Pharmaceutical Committee (2015). *Overview of Member States Biennial Reports on Audits of their Pharmacovigilance Systems (2013 Reporting Year)*. Pharmaceutical Committee, 21 October 2015, PHARM 693.

European Commission (2016). *Pharmacovigilance Related Activities of Member States and the European Medicines Agency Concerning Medicinal Products for Human Use (2012-2014)*, COM(2016) 498 final, Brussels, 08.08.2016.

Jadeja, M., Barrow, P. (2016). *Topic 4.3: Awareness Levels*. SCOPE Work Package 4 Survey Report.

Jan, T., Radecka, (2015). *Topic 4 Review of Reporting Forms*. SCOPE Work Package 4 Survey Report.

Klein, K., De Bruin, M. L., Broekmans, A. W., Stolk, P. (2015*). Classification of Recombinant Biologics in the EU: Divergence between National Pharmacovigilance Centres*. BioDrugs 29: 373-379.

Moore, N., Bégaud, B. (2010). *Improving Pharmacovigilance in Europe*. The BMJ 340: c1694.

Šarinić, V. M., Di Giusti, M. D., Banovac, M., Skurce, N. M., Gvozdanović, K., Krnic, D., Andrić, A., Šipić, I., Cajko, N., Sudić, D., Lovretić, N. (2016). *Topic 1 Audit of National Reporting Systems, Topic 1a Medication Errors, Topic 2 Patient Reporting, Topic 5 Review of IT Systems and Special Form of Reports*. SCOPE Work Package 4 Survey Report.

Vermeer, N. S., Straus, S. M. J. M., Mantel-Teeuwisse, A. K., Domergue, F., Egberts, T. C. G., Leufkens, H. G. M., De Bruin, M. L. (2013). *Traceability of Biopharmaceuticals in Spontaneous Reporting Systems: A Cross-Sectional Study in the FDA Adverse Event Reporting System (FAERS) and EudraVigilance Databases*. Drug Safety 36: 617-625.

Vermeer, N. S., Spierings, I., Mantel-Teeuwisse, A. K., Straus, S. M. J. M., Giezen, T. J., Leufkens, H. G. M., Egberts, T. C. G., De Bruin, M. L. (2015). *Traceability of Biologicals: Present Challenges in Pharmacovigilance*. Expert Opinion on Drug Safety, 14 (1).

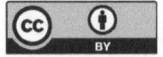

Conclusions and Recommendations 7

Pharmacovigilance is vital for public health and patient safety and includes all activities relating to the detection, assessment and prevention of adverse effects due to medicinal products (see WHO 2004). Despite risk assessment before marketing authorisation, all medicines might produce adverse drug reactions (ADRs) during therapeutic use after marketing (Belton and the European Pharmacovigilance Research Group 1997).

Overall, the findings of our comparative assessment of six national pharmacovigilance systems for biological medicinal products (biologicals) are rich and encouraging, yet somehow sobering. The in-depth analysis includes six important aims corresponding to the structure of the manuscript.

Chapter 2 illustrates that because all medicines might produce ADRs, timely and accurate reporting is important to ensure post-market authorisation safety. Due to their intrinsic characteristics, this is particularly true regarding biologicals.

Chapter 3 illustrates that the EU pharmaceuticals regulation was mainly concerned with pre-market authorisation up until the 1990s, whereas pharmacovigilance was rather neglected. Since that time, pharmacovigilance has begun to become an important aspect of EU regulation. The system of pharmacovigilance has been substantially reformed with the adoption of Directive 2010/84/EU, which amended Directive 2001/83/EC. Today, extended provisions for Member States to establish national pharmacovigilance systems are in place through Article 102 of Directive 2010/84/EU.

Chapter 4 stresses, however, that many countries have a serious transposition problem in their national pharmacovigilance systems. Almost 85 percent of the national transposition instruments are not transposed on time, and in fact are delayed up to more than two years.

Chapter 5 takes into account the various types of national public health systems and presents different perceived challenges and best practices for each Member

State; the variation in national public health corresponds with the variation in national pharmacovigilance systems.

Chapter 6 focuses on the core finding which is ADR underreporting. Based on our research methodology involving desk and field research, we have compared the major challenges and identified individual as well as organisational factors impeding appropriate ADR reporting.

Notwithstanding the recorded progress across Member States, the reform of the EU pharmacovigilance system could be further improved. Important challenges remain regarding both legal transposition and practical implementation across Europe. Drawing on these challenges, this chapter describes a list of recommendations with a view to improving practical implementation in the Member States. In order to facilitate a better understanding among Member States, identified best practices based on the comparative analysis are included as well.

The first part describes specific recommendations structured along Article 102 of Directive 2010/84/EU. The article specifies the general provisions on pharmacovigilance and lays down a number of measures regarding ADR reporting. We concentrate on the role of healthcare providers because Article 102 further specifies that for the purposes of points (a) and (e) of the first paragraph the Member States may impose specific obligations on doctors, pharmacists and other healthcare professionals.

In the second part, more general recommendations are derived from the specific measures regarding ADR reporting. These general recommendations have to be understood in the context of different ideal systems of national healthcare.

7.1   Specific Recommendations in Relation to Article 102

In accordance with Article 102, the Member States shall:

a. take all appropriate measures to encourage patients, doctors, pharmacists and other healthcare professionals to report suspected adverse reactions to the national competent authority; for these tasks, organisations representing consumers, patients and healthcare professionals may be involved as appropriate;

This provision is a cornerstone of the pharmacovigilance reform, because it includes for the first time patients as actors in national pharmacovigilance systems. However, the analysis revealed that patients lack awareness regarding their role in pharmacovigilance and therefore often do not report ADRs.

- **Recommendation 1**: In order to tackle underreporting by patients, European, national and regional authorities should invest in awareness-raising campaigns to increase the public knowledge about pharmacovigilance and ADR reporting.
- **Recommendation 2**: Authorities should raise awareness in the short term through various means of communication, e.g. websites, social media, leaflets (best practice: Poland, the United Kingdom) as well as in the long term through cooperation with schools to educate future generations (best practice: Portugal).

Although doctors, pharmacists and other healthcare providers are "classic" actors in pharmacovigilance, the analysis also revealed that the problem of underreporting is still prevalent. For a number of reasons, healthcare professionals often do not report ADRs.

- **Recommendation 3:** In order to tackle underreporting by healthcare providers, national authorities and healthcare institutions should invest in awareness-raising campaigns to increase professional knowledge about pharmacovigilance and sensitise relevant actors about its particular importance to ensure public health.

In the analysis, a distinction was made between quantity (number of ADR reports) and quality (value of information in ADR reports). While awareness-raising campaigns are expected to increase quantity, additional measures need to be implemented to increase the quality of ADR reporting as well.

- **Recommendation 4:** In order to improve both the quantity and quality of ADR reports, university classes about the importance of pharmacovigilance and the need for ADR reporting should be mandatory for every medical and pharmacy student (best practice: Finland).
- **Recommendation 5:** In addition, European, national or regional authorities should organise advanced post-graduate training on a regular basis to ensure that healthcare professionals acquire the necessary skills for coping with the complex task of ADR reporting.[8]
- **Recommendation 6:** Healthcare professionals should also be trained to encourage patients to report and to assist them, if needed, with high-quality reporting.

---

8   Such training should include practical and legal counseling in order to alleviate the fear of litigation. However, this recommendation is contingent on the national legal system in which ADR reporting occurs (see below).

Because healthcare providers working in healthcare institutions are not isolated actors, institutional factors contribute to the effective implementation of pharmacovigilance measures. The analysis revealed a number of challenges in this respect. For instance, ADR reporting is often perceived to be time-consuming and incompatible with other tasks.

- **Recommendation 7:** Healthcare institutions, in line with the general health policies of their Member State, should facilitate ADR reporting through streamlined internal processes.
- **Recommendation 8:** All stakeholders at the national level should improve mechanisms of cooperation. This not only includes competent authorities, but also industry and patients' associations as well as research and training facilities such as universities.

b. facilitate patient reporting through the provision of alternative reporting formats in addition to web-based formats;

Because the reform of the pharmacovigilance system includes patients for the first time, a related stipulation was included to facilitate patient reporting through alternative formats. Despite these formats, the analysis revealed that formatting adds to the challenges regarding patients' reporting.

- **Recommendation 9:** In order to facilitate ADR reporting for patients, Member States should offer a wide range of possible communication channels, including web-based and paper-based formats.
- **Recommendation 10:** Both web-based and paper-based formats should be designed to be as user-friendly as possible. For web-based formats, IT solutions should be developed to guide patients through the format and to ensure the completeness of reports. All formats should be accompanied by accessible manuals written in layman's terms.

SCOPE data indicates that user-friendly formatting helps increase ADR reporting by patients (Jan, Radecka 2015: 63-64). Hence, in order to follow up on these recommendations, Member States should engage in mutual learning and sharing of best practices within the framework of SCOPE or otherwise.

c. take all appropriate measures to obtain accurate and verifiable data for the scientific evaluation of suspected adverse reaction reports;

This provision is relevant insofar as it indicates the importance of scientific evaluation of individual reports regarding assessing the causality of a drug and the related ADR(s). The analysis revealed that often information is not available due to technical reasons, for instance when databases are not compatible.

- **Recommendation 11:** In order to cope with information overload and to facilitate the process of submitting ADR reports, national and regional competent authorities should improve interconnectivity of IT systems, such as for instance those of general practitioners, hospitals, pharmacies and the national competent authority's ADR reporting system (best practice: United Kingdom).
- **Recommendation 12:** In addition to measures for facilitating patient reporting, national and regional competent authorities should also establish mechanisms to provide mandatory feedback to reporting patients.

d. ensure that the public is given important information on pharmacovigilance concerns relating to the use of a medicinal product in a timely manner through publication on the web-portal and through other means of publicly available information as necessary;

As mentioned in Chapter 3, this stipulation was included through an amendment of the European Parliament (EP) during the legislative process leading to the adoption of Directive 2010/84/EU. Drawing on the precautionary principle, the inclusion is geared towards dissemination of information to healthcare professionals and patients.

Drawing on the comparative analysis and the various recommendations dealing with other stipulations of Article 102, we can provide a general recommendation in this respect.

- **Recommendation 13:** With a view to effective communication of pharmacovigilance information to patients, stakeholders at the national and European level should build on existing mechanisms of cooperation and should strive to build additional mechanisms in line with the means applied for raising general awareness of pharmacovigilance (best practice: Germany).

e. ensure, through the methods for collecting information and where necessary
   through the follow-up of suspected adverse reaction reports, that all appropriate
   measures are taken to identify clearly any biological medicinal product prescribed, dispensed or sold in their territory which is the subject of a suspected
   adverse reaction report, with due regard to the name of the medicinal product,
   in accordance with Article 1(20), and the batch number;

This provision is of particular relevance regarding the traceability of biologicals.
The analysis revealed that the practices of ADR reporting in the Member States
do not ensure traceability throughout. Across Member States, batch numbers are
not recorded by healthcare professionals as a routine task. Because biologicals are
a special case of general ADR reporting, similar recommendations can be derived.

- **Recommendation 14:** In order to tackle underreporting of batch numbers and
  thereby facilitate the correct and timely traceability of biologicals, healthcare
  professionals should receive additional training to both increase awareness about
  the particular relevance of ADR reporting related to biologicals and to acquire
  the necessary skills to do so (best practice: Finland).
- **Recommendation 15:** Healthcare institutions, in line with the general health
  policies of their Member State, should facilitate ADR reporting through streamlined internal processes and improved mechanisms of cooperation.

7.2   General Recommendations: National Healthcare Systems and Policy Options for Pharmacovigilance

Drawing on the specific recommendations in relation to Article 102, we have developed general recommendations in the context of 1) the individual level of healthcare
providers reporting ADRs; 2) the organisational level of healthcare institutions that
provide for the environment in which healthcare professionals fulfil their tasks;
and 3) the systemic level of pharmacovigilance in the Member States.

Individual Level of Healthcare Providers Reporting ADRs

Our analysis revealed that in some countries, medical liability presents an important
impediment to ADR reporting by healthcare professionals. However, the fear of
medical liability is contingent on the national health policy and the legal system
on which it is based.

In general, there are two systems of compensation for patients that have suffered from medical injuries (see Simon and Jansen 2009). On the one hand, so-called no-fault systems provide compensation through national healthcare services. On the other hand, private healthcare providers or even individual healthcare professionals can be held liable. Hence, no-fault systems are usually associated with healthcare systems in which states are the main providers of health services and claims made by patients are made directly with them (see Romeo-Casabona 2009). In our sample, France, for instance, has a no-fault system, whereas Portugal and Germany have fault-based models (Essinger 2009).[9]

In this respect, the Council of Europe put forward a number of recommendations to improve patient safety and prevent adverse events in healthcare (Council of Europe 2009). Regarding ADR reporting, the recommendations are very similar to the provisions enshrined in Article 102 of Directive 2010/84/EU. However, the recommendations are based on a no-fault approach in which patients' rights ought to be accommodated with the requirements of extensive ADR reporting. Therefore, the recommendations include that legal protection of reporting healthcare professionals ought to be ensured.

During the reform of the EU pharmacovigilance system, the European Parliament aimed to include the same approach by amending Article 102, stating that "reporting of suspected adverse reactions due to medication errors should be on a 'no blame' basis, and should be legally privileged" (European Parliament 2010).

Due to the diversity of national health systems, it is not surprising that this amendment was rejected by Member States. Its inclusion would imply a total overhaul of established legal principles going beyond pharmacovigilance.

- **Recommendation on the individual level of healthcare providers reporting ADRs**: However, taking into account national diversity in health-related and legal terms, it is important to recognise that fault-based systems are an important impediment for ADR reporting. A general and cautious recommendation would then call on the Member States to enable healthcare professionals to report ADRs without fear of liability. This could be pursued not only by practical and legal counselling for healthcare professionals, but also by legal means through strengthening confidentiality or setting up compensation schemes for patients' claims.

---

9   However, simple categorisations cannot be made because the issue of patients' claims and compensations is a highly complex legal issue (see Romeo-Casabona 2009).

Organisational Level of Healthcare Institutions That Provide for the Environment in Which Healthcare Professionals Fulfil Their Tasks

Our analysis revealed that in many countries, the reporting of an ADR is perceived as admitting a failure. Therefore, healthcare professionals may decide not to report.

Regarding the implementation of Article 102, we have derived a specific recommendation calling for awareness-raising campaigns to increase professional knowledge about pharmacovigilance. While such campaigns are important for healthcare professionals in order to be aware of ADR reporting, this general recommendation points to a broader problem at the institutional level.

At this level, the behaviour of individuals is affected by institutional norms and values. That ADRs are seen as failures is one such value. Another one is the perceived loss of reputation. These norms and values cannot be changed by creating incentives at the individual level. Instead, national policy makers, healthcare providers and hospital management are called on to introduce a different culture of care and patient safety in which ADR reporting is seen as a key responsibility of healthcare professionals.

This general recommendation, however, has to be qualified by stressing that there are different corporate cultures in national institutions of healthcare provisions. The example of Finland is a case in point; hospitals in Finland are run based on strict hierarchical structures. On the one hand, change can be more easily implemented from top to bottom in this kind of organisation. If, on the other hand, top management is resistant to change, a hierarchical organisation increases the chance of resistance from healthcare professionals in their day-to-day work.

- **Recommendation on the organisation level of healthcare institutions that provide for the environment in which healthcare professionals fulfil their tasks:** By all means, pharmacovigilance should receive a more prominent role in the education of healthcare professionals, be they doctors, pharmacists or nursing staff. Cultural changes at the institutional level in hospitals and other healthcare providers can only be internalised by healthcare professionals if the underlying values and benefits of ADR reporting are included in the curricula of universities and other training facilities. Such long-term strategies are essential to affect the "corporate" culture in the healthcare institutions of the Member States.

Systemic Level of Pharmacovigilance in Member States

Several of our respondents considered a high level of collaboration between the relevant actors to be particularly beneficial for the process of ADR reporting. Thus, as a general recommendation, Member States can be called on to improve cooperation among all actors in the national pharmacovigilance systems. The underlying assumption here is that inclusive systems are an important precondition for the effective implementation of ADR reporting.

This recommendation, however, has to be qualified by stressing the diversity of national systems. Some Member States have centralised systems of pharmacovigilance, and others have de-centralised systems. Some Member States have separate systems for biologicals, while others do not. Calls for further cooperation thus have to take into account the institutional structure of healthcare providers and the respective corporate cultures.

Whereas Portugal, for instance, has introduced regional centres after initially establishing a centralised system, this option might not be available for all Member States. Germany, for example, has a centralised system. Yet sectoral associations provide functional links between patients, healthcare providers and national competent authorities.

In general, subsidiarity is a key concept here. Challenges for national pharmacovigilance systems, which should be addressed in the short term, e.g. training and awareness raising, should be devised in line with existing systemic features of national health systems. Long-term strategies require substantial reform of these systems and go beyond the implementation of the EU pharmacovigilance system.

A case in point is the particular challenge of the German pharmacovigilance system. Here, data protection is an important impediment. Some Member States have impeding policies in place which are entrenched in the national political culture and which cannot be changed easily. After all, such changes require trade-offs of competing policy objectives at the EU level and, even more important, at the national level.

Another case in point of system-level impediment is the economic crisis. As could be seen in the various country chapters, the scarcity of resources more or less affects all Member States. However, the problem is particularly acute in Southern European Member States such as Portugal, where the national pharmacovigilance system is only slowly recovering from the deep financial and personnel cuts in the recent years. By all means, the scarcity of financial and human resources has to be seen as a structural factor regarding the regulation of complex policy issues, of which pharmaceuticals policy is just one.

- **Recommendation on the systemic level of pharmacovigilance in the Member States:** In general, national and regional competent authorities working under the auspices of national ministries should be endowed with sufficient financial means to fulfil their functions. Likewise, healthcare institutions should be endowed with sufficient means. Sound finances enable healthcare institutions to rely on a stronger workforce which reduces the workload of individual healthcare professionals and increases the possibility of extended ADR reporting.

References

Belton, K. J. and the European Pharmacovigilance Group (1997). *Attitude Survey of Adverse Drug-Reaction Reporting by Health Care Professionals across the European Union*. European Journal of Pharmacology 52: 423-427.

Council of Europe (2009). *The Ever-Growing Challenge of Medical Liability: National and European Responses*. Strasbourg, 2-3 June 2009, Conference Proceedings.

Essinger, K. (2009). Medical Liability: Alternative Ways to Court Procedures. Council of Europe (ed) (2009). *The Ever-Growing Challenge of Medical Liability: National and European Responses*. Strasbourg, 2-3 June 2009, Conference Proceedings.

Romeo-Casabona, C. (2009). The Legal Approach to Medical Liability – Negligence and Breach of Patient's Autonomy. Council of Europe (ed) (2009). *The Ever-Growing Challenge of Medical Liability: National and European Responses*. Strasbourg, 2-3 June 2009, Conference Proceedings.

Simon, J., Jansen, B. (2009). Economic Implications of Medical Liability Claims: Insurance and Compensation Schemes. Council of Europe (ed) (2009). *The Ever-Growing Challenge of Medical Liability: National and European Responses*. Strasbourg, 2-3 June 2009, Conference Proceedings.

WHO (2004). *Pharmacovigilance: Ensuring the Safe Use of Medicines*. WHO Policy Perspectives on Medicines 9.

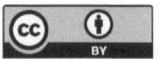